DO Y[illegible]
H[illegible]

Are you su[illegible] y, loss of attention, “fuzzy” thinking? Do you have hearing problems, skin rashes, persistent coughs, mysterious allergies? It may not be “just in your head.” Each year 390,000 workers suffer some job-related illness or injury. *Your* symptoms may have an occupational source. Discover what’s really wrong and how to fix it. Learn:

- How to minimize the daily stress of your job
- What you can do to prevent work-related hearing loss
- The seven factors in the workplace that result in psychological disorders and how to change them
- What they don’t tell you about occupationally induced skin disease and what you can do to protect yourself

Everything you need to know is here. There are no more excuses. What you do *now* could change your life.

WHY IS THIS JOB KILLING ME?
Read it. It’s good for you.

For Anne — Good luck in Florida — we'll miss you!

Why Is This Job Killing Me?

John & Mary

John B. Kachuba and
Mary A. Newman, Ph.D., CIH

A Dell Book

Published by
Dell Publishing
a division of
Random House, Inc.
1540 Broadway
New York, New York 10036

Dell books may be purchased for business or promotional use or for special sales. For information please write to: Special Markets Department, Random House, Inc., 1540 Broadway, New York, N.Y. 10036

ISBN: 0-440-23486-7

Designed by Sabrina Bowers

Printed in the United States of America

Published simultaneously in Canada

July 1999

10 9 8 7 6 5 4 3 2 1

OPM

This book is dedicated to our children—
Amy, Kristen, Jeff, Sarah, and Matt—
may they always work in a safe and
healthful environment

Authors' Note

A portion of our profits from this book will be donated to the Alice Hamilton Foundation.

Dr. Alice Hamilton (1869–1970) was a pioneer in the field of industrial hygiene in the United States and is sometimes called the Mother of Industrial Hygiene. A tireless physician and social reformer, she spent much of her early years at Jane Addams' Hull House in Chicago, engaged in social and medical issues. Trained in pathology and bacteriology, Dr. Hamilton served as chief investigator on the Illinois Occupational Disease Commission's survey of occupational health problems in 1910, the first survey of its kind in this country. In 1919, Dr. Hamilton became the first woman appointed to the faculty at Harvard University, teaching industrial hygiene there part of each year, while working in her own area of scientific inquiry the remainder of the time. The recipient of numerous international awards, Dr. Hamilton wrote *Exploring the Dangerous Trades* when she was in her seventies.

The Alice Hamilton Foundation is dedicated to creating awareness of occupational safety and health issues worldwide and seeks to work especially with underserved populations such as women, minorities, and developing nations.

Contents

Preface

When I was a boy, my uncle told me about the canary. On a tour of the abandoned Pennsylvania coal mine in which he had spent most of his working life, he told me that when the canary stopped singing it was time to get out of the mine.

Anyone who has ever owned a canary knows that the little birds are nonstop singers. Coal miners used to take a canary with them down into the mines. If dangerously explosive gases were present in the mine, their fumes killed the bird and silenced his song. The miners were warned by the silence that their own lives were in danger.

Miners no longer use canaries. Modern technology has provided more sophisticated warning systems. Yet, accidents still occur. Carelessness, lack of training, physical exhaustion, cost-cutting, defective equipment, and improper work practices are some of the factors that contribute to occupational injuries and illnesses in mines and many other industries. Millions of Americans suffer from job-related illnesses or accidents.

I know what you're thinking. "What has this got to do with me? I don't even *know* a miner."

There are many high-risk jobs that can cause injuries and death besides mining. Logging, fishing, construction, farming, and fire fighting are just a few. But you don't have to be employed in high-risk jobs to experience occupational accidents and diseases.

Secretaries, computer operators, writers, musicians, and assembly line workers may suffer from carpal tunnel syndrome—a painful disorder of the wrist caused by repetitive motions and correctable only through surgery. Teachers, office workers, and store clerks are sometimes inflicted with headaches, allergies, and asthma caused by poor indoor air quality. Painters and factory workers may suffer from headaches or depression as a result of their use of solvents, cleaners, and degreasers. Some of these materials may also cause cancer. Doctors, nurses, aides, and other hospital workers are daily at risk of contracting hepatitis, AIDS, and other infectious diseases. Sales and customer service workers strain their eyes watching video display terminals all day. Even salesmen, talking on cellular car phones, may be at some risk of developing cancer of the brain caused by electromagnetic radiation. The same may be true for police officers using handheld radar detectors.

In short, *anyone* who works for a living is risking his good health, perhaps his life, because of job-related illnesses and injuries.

There is no reason why millions of Americans each year should become ill or injured on the job. The risk to our health and well-being, caused by an unsafe workplace, is something we have come to take for granted, believing that the conditions cannot change, that's just the way it is.

We have been lulled by our own ignorance and the interests of corporate profitability into a sense of false security about the workplace. We believe it is handguns, crime in the streets, auto accidents, high-cholesterol diets that will do us in, not our jobs.

The canaries would sing the truth. They would tell us

that we have to take responsibility for the 56,000 Americans who will die this year from job-related accidents or illnesses. Many more will be injured, maimed, or left with the seed of a fatal disease growing within them.

Where are the canaries? Who will warn us?

JOHN B. KACHUBA

CHAPTER 1

Introduction

The Invisible Environment

Every nine minutes, someone is killed by their job.

A little quick math and that number translates into 56,000 deaths each year, almost as many deaths in one year as the number of American fatalities in Vietnam throughout the war's duration. In 1994, employers reported 6.3 million disabling work injuries and 515,000 cases of occupational disease.[1]

Americans today are very health conscious. We try to improve our health by dieting and exercise, by giving up tobacco and alcohol, and by reducing our cholesterol levels and blood pressure, but we pay little attention to substances and activities at our jobs that can kill us outright or deliver us a slow, lingering death. Worst of all, we do not even recognize these silent killers.

We know how poorly or well we treat our bodies and we understand the dangers to our health caused by pollution and the destruction of our natural environment. We read about the threat to virgin forests and the spotted owl, wetlands and manatees, and we do what we can to help. We donate money or join the Sierra Club, the Nature Conservancy, or any one of hundreds of organizations dedicated to saving our natural environment and natural resources. We mobilize in grassroots groups to stop local threats to the environment, such as unwanted toxic waste sites, oil pipelines, dams, and the desecration of wilderness areas. We do all these things because we understand that a poisoned environment will poison us. But we ignore our workplace environment.

Even those experts who should be warning us about workplace hazards remain dangerously ignorant of them. Environmentalists easily recognize hazards to plants and animals caused by soil erosion, air and water pollution, and deforestation. They blame industry for much of this damage yet they seem unable to include the workplace environment in a broader definition of "environment." They see industrial pollutants pouring into rivers, leaving fish belly-up, but they fail to see the many workers, exposed to these same pollutants on the job, who will die or suffer serious health consequences as a result of their exposures.

They do not see the thousands who will be stricken with respiratory diseases, cancer, neurological diseases, reproductive disorders, and a host of other ailments simply as a result of working. There is an interconnectedness between the natural and workplace environments that must be put into perspective. The interconnectedness lies in the fact that we cannot separate our lives neatly into one environment or the other. What we do at our jobs, the pollutants and destruction that we create through our work, will have a damaging impact upon the natural environment that boomerangs back to us in the form of serious health effects caused by poisoned air and water, pesticide-sprayed fruits and vegetables, depletion of the ozone layer, and a host of other ailments. Controls must remain in place to protect our natural environment from industrial damage, not only to protect our plant and animal life, but to protect *our* lives.

The disasters at Bhopal and Chernobyl, in which thousands died, left behind many more with serious health effects, and the surrounding countryside was contaminated, never to be used again. These serve as tragic examples of industrial destruction. They remind us that what goes wrong in our workplace environment can destroy the natural environment and surrounding communities as well. Occupational safety and health must become the concern of everyone.

But we must understand that the greatest risk to our health occurs every day, in the workplace. We do not need tragic, headline-making accidents in order to become a victim of an unsafe workplace. In most cases, toxins in the workplace are insidious, nibbling away at our health bit by bit. Frequently, we do not find out what is happening to us until it is too late. Sometimes we never find out at all.

What You Don't Know

What you don't know about your workplace could kill you. Most of us really do not understand the safety and health risks associated with our jobs. Sure, it's easy to see the dangers that firefighters, policemen, steelworkers, miners, and others face each day, but what about the rest of us? What about factory workers, store clerks, painters, nurses, office workers? What about dry cleaners, dentists, mechanics, morticians? It is difficult to find an occupation that does not have some health risks attached to it. Yet we remain ignorant of these risks, an ignorance that is quite literally killing us. Our lack of knowledge is caused by several factors:

- **Lack of education**—Our formal education does not include learning about workplace hazards. Occupational safety and health issues are not included as part of health or science courses. Even vocational training rarely educates students about occupational diseases or injuries common to the workplace. It's likely that teachers themselves do not know enough about these matters to teach others. Or, it may be that teachers do not wish to discourage students from entering certain occupational fields by discussing the negative aspects of some jobs. In either case, the result is the same: we do not learn about workplace hazards that may affect our health.

The educational system is failing to teach students about occupational safety and health and is falling ever farther behind. The world is changing fast. New technologies result in new hazards introduced to the workplace almost daily. Some examples:

"Ergonomics," the term for the technology that makes machines safer and "user friendly," could not be found in dictionaries before 1960. Today, automobile interiors are designed to be "ergonomically correct," as are office furnishings and workstation equipment. Entire books are written about carpal tunnel syndrome, an ergonomic disorder resulting in painfully pinched nerves of the wrist that requires surgical correction. The largest fine ever proposed by the Occupational Safety and Health Administration (OSHA), originally $4.3 million, was against John Morrell & Co. for repetitive motion injuries, carpal tunnel syndrome.[2]

A rash of cancer deaths among police officers have led some researchers to believe that there may be a link between cancer of the brain and new applications of electromagnetic radiation, such as radar guns and cellular phones.

The new technology of irradiating foods to kill bacteria has some scientists worried about the effects of radiation on food processors and consumers.

The list goes on. New threats to our health and safety in the workplace are appearing every day.

- **Lack of training**—Frequently, employers do not provide adequate on-the-job training about safety and health hazards found in their workplaces. As a result, more than half of all occupational injuries occur to employees with less than one year's experience on the job.[3] Despite the fact that there is an OSHA regulation, known as the Hazard Communication Standard, already in place that requires employers to provide full disclosure on any and all safety and health hazards in their particular workplace, full disclosure is either glossed over, given to us in an edited fashion, or omitted entirely.

  It's not unusual for some businesses to edit this information in order to create the appearance of a safe workplace. Although this edited disclosure violates the Hazard Communication Standard, unscrupulous businesses can find a way around the standard by claiming that full disclosure of safety and health effects would also reveal confidential proprietary information of value to competitors. The result is that workers end up handling a witch's brew of chemicals labeled ambiguously as "solvents," "cleaners," and "disinfectants" without ever knowing the actual chemical components to which they are exposed.

  In a few cases, companies are aware of the health hazards relative to their business but deliberately choose to violate the law and keep their employees in the dark. With OSHA enforcement as lax as it is, these companies are infrequently brought to justice.

  Most businesses have the good intention of providing full disclosure but cannot do an adequate job of it because they cannot afford to hire knowledgeable safety and health personnel to provide worker training or industrial hygienists to investigate hazards. Or, it may be that they do not understand the workplace hazards themselves. These companies roll the dice and hope their business will not be inspected by OSHA, or if they are inspected and found deficient in some areas, that they would be penalized only a moderate fine. Unfortunately for the workers involved, this gamble often pays off for the company.

In many cases, it's a matter of the fox guarding the henhouse, since each business and industry is solely responsible for the training and education of its employees. There is no independent, unbiased source available for worker training in occupational hazards.

- **Worker perceptions**—Even when workers suspect that their health problems are workplace induced they may not know what to do about them. Faced with confusing reporting systems, and unsure of the cause of their symptoms, workers sometimes decide that doing nothing at all is the best course.

  Many workers believe that health hazards come with the territory, that they have always been a part of the job and always will be. They have heard so many exaggerated reports about substances that may be carcinogens—everything from the preservatives used in nail polish to peanut butter—that the common belief is that everything causes cancer. It can't be avoided. This jaded attitude blinds workers to the true hazards common to their job. As an example, the media attention that has been given to AIDS in the last few years roused labor unions to lobby OSHA for a standard. In response, OSHA issued the Bloodborne Disease Standard, which also included regulations for other contagious diseases such as hepatitis. Although hepatitis kills far more health care workers each year than AIDS, the unions had failed to recognize the hepatitis threat and pushed for legal guidelines only when the notorious AIDS virus entered the picture.

With such distorted perceptions, workers are frequently uninformed about unsafe workplaces or given incorrect information. Unless workers become truly knowledgeable about the situation, change never happens.

Some workers fear that any complaints about their workplace environment could cost them their jobs or worse, as the speculation about the death of Karen Silkwood would imply. Whistle-blowers have not been immune to retaliation from their employers. Helpless in unsettled economic times as ours, some workers would rather work in an unsafe environment than not work at all.

- **Delayed health effects**—Many occupational diseases go unreported because their effects occur much later in life and it is difficult to make a cause-and-effect link at that time. Still, we know that a large number of health problems, such as cancer, miscarriages (spontaneous abortions), impotence, and respiratory diseases such as asthma may be related to workplace hazards. This is also true for a wide variety of lesser ailments such as headaches, nausea, dermatitis, and fatigue.

  Many deaths due to occupational factors may occur 10, 15, 20 years after exposure. Lung disease and several types of cancers proceed this way. When the worker finally succumbs to his disease, the true cause of death may not be clearly linked to the workplace, especially if the worker also smoked, drank alcohol, or had a history of other medical conditions. Any of these existing health problems could have been made worse by an occupational disease. When the true cause of death is misdiagnosed, the myth of a safe workplace is perpetuated.

We are unable to protect ourselves against these types of occupational diseases because of their insidious onset and our ignorance of workplace hazards. Consequently, we wait too long to take action. This is especially true in diseases of the reproductive system. By the time a woman actually becomes pregnant, and concerned about the health of her unborn child, she may have already been exposed to high levels of dangerous chemicals or other hazards that may result in a spontaneous abortion or the birth of a child with serious health effects.

- **Corporate collusion**—Another reason why our knowledge of occupational safety and health issues is weak can be traced to the role of some businesses in subverting any regulatory measures that affect profits. These businesses are reluctant to spend money on any changes that may be required by safety and health regulations. The cost of implementation of such regulations always seems too expensive for them to remain competitive. Business leaders threaten layoffs and plant closings if their cost of operations is increased by safety regulations. The now defunct Council on Competitiveness, set up by former Vice President Dan Quayle, repeatedly helped businesses find loopholes in regulations, generally pertaining to environmental and health and safety issues, in order for economic growth to continue unimpeded. This growth-above-all view is often myopic since the cost of medical care, insurance, wage losses, and administration, all of which are the result of inadequate safety and health policies, can total into the billions of dollars, \$130.7 billion in 1997, according to the National Safety

Council, $358 million a day.[4] Still, with many businesses carefully eyeing profits on a day-to-day basis, corporate attorneys are kept busy inventing methods of stalling or circumventing health and safety regulations.

Business also has a direct influence on new regulations being proposed by OSHA. As a result of Executive Order 12291, signed by President Reagan in 1981, the Office of Management and Budget (OMB) was required to review all regulations developed by federal agencies and apply a dehumanizing cost-benefit analysis to them. Now, when a new regulation is proposed OSHA solicits testimony from business leaders to assess what the cost of implementation of the new regulation would be to the businesses involved. Some businesses will grossly inflate the cost estimate they give to OSHA. The agency then arrives at a cost-benefit calculation in which they determine exactly how many deaths in the workplace are "acceptable," based on the cost of implementation of the new regulations. Since their calculations are often based upon deliberately inaccurate information provided by business, the number of actual deaths is much higher than it should be. Going beyond the OSHA system, there are many who argue that one single workplace death is not "acceptable."

Corporations are sometimes assisted in skirting regulations by politicians and lobbyists. In 1992, President Bush declared a three-month moratorium on any new OSHA regulations, ostensibly to spur a lagging economy. At the end of three months, he extended the moratorium an additional four months. The administration claimed that the freeze on regulations would allow businesses the chance to "catch up" in a weak economy and would save them $10 to $20 billion dollars. Public interest groups such as OMB Watch and Ralph Nader's Public Citizen claimed that the moratorium was responsible for 293 deaths and more than 1.3 million injuries in its first 90 days of implementation.[5]

- **Government weakness**—Another reason why workers are unaware of occupational safety and health hazards is that both federal and state governments lack the funding and resources necessary to promote awareness of existing regulations, enforce existing regulations, and develop new ones.

The annual budget allocated to OSHA to protect a workforce of 100 million workers is $380 million, a paltry sum of $3.11 per worker, per year, less than one hour's minimum wage.[6]

The minuscule OSHA budget restricts the agency's ability to develop adequate safety and health training programs and to effectively fill the needs of business. It also means that there are not nearly enough OSHA inspectors available to police the millions of workplaces in this country, leaving them effectively self-policed. Following the 1991 Imperial Foods fire in North Carolina, in which 25 workers were killed, the media reported that the facility had not been inspected by OSHA for several years. This should not have come as a surprise, since 924 OSHA inspectors are expected to perform inspections of 7 million work sites. At that rate, OSHA can inspect workplaces on an average of once every 109 years.

The same limitations apply to the National Institute for Occupational Safety and Health (NIOSH). This agency is research oriented, seeking to uncover occupational safety and health hazards and recommending methods of recognizing, evaluating, and controlling them. NIOSH, also underfunded and understaffed, can only work on a small fraction of the total number of health hazards afflicting our workplace environment.

- **Media disregard**—Except in rare cases, the media simply does not report on worker safety-and-health issues. They will report every airplane crash, every earthquake, hurricane, tornado, flood, and California brushfire that may result in the loss of human life, but the media gives short shrift to occupational illnesses and accidents. Only spectacular disasters such as the tragic construction accident at L'Ambiance Plaza in Bridgeport, Connecticut, that killed 28 workers, or the fire at Imperial Foods in North Carolina, in which twenty-five workers perished, seem to get media attention.

Effecting a Change

What can be done to guarantee the health and safety of America's workforce?

We must first understand how dangerous are our workplaces. We must also understand that we have an undeniable right to a healthful workplace. Companies must be prevailed upon, through a combination of moral persuasion, legal enforcement, and good business sense, to provide a safer and more healthful workplace environment.

Knowledge is power, the power necessary for us to take control of our lives in the workplace. In order to create a safe and healthy workplace environment we must learn all that we can about our jobs, the equipment used, the chemicals to which we may be exposed, and mechanical hazards that may exist on the job.

Litigation involving stronger penalties and criminal liability for individuals, as well as corporations, may help to enforce existing occupational safety and health laws, but it is not enough to solve the problem. Greater attention must be focused on new regulations, especially as our technology advances and new safety and health hazards are introduced almost daily into the workplace environment.

Environmental regulations have already been enacted, such as the Clean Air Act, that are designed to reduce the amount of toxic materials that industries are allowed to spew into the air and water. While they afford some protection to the natural environment, these regulations do little to protect the health and safety of workers who must still handle these materials in their toxic state, before expulsion from the site. Stronger regulations are needed to reduce the hazards we face at our job sites. These regulations may require the replacement of dangerous chemicals with other nontoxic substances, or may call for design and engineering changes within the facility or with the equipment being used. Some may even call for a change in a manufacturing process. Whatever their specifics, the emphasis of future regulations must shift to worker protection.

The shift to worker protection could have far-reaching consequences for the community. The Resource Conservation and Recovery Act (RCRA) and the Comprehensive Environmental Response, Compensation, and Liability Act (CERCLA) already regulate the reporting of industrial spills and releases of hazardous wastes and materials to community and government agencies. This enables the community to take the timely actions needed to protect its citizens in time of emergency. Creating stronger regulations to protect workers on the job would greatly reduce the occurrence of accidents that could affect the community, thus safeguarding both individuals and the community at large.

It all comes down to this: We are responsible for our own health and safety in the workplace. Just as we can make a conscious decision to stop smoking or drinking, or to go on a diet or exercise more often, we can decide to create safer workplace environments. That is a decision we can make. It is a decision we *must* make.

References

1. National Institute for Occupational Safety and Health (NIOSH). 1997. *New Directions at NIOSH*. Cincinnati: NIOSH.
2. Mokhiber, Russell. 1989. *Corporate Crime and Violence: Big Business and the Abuse of the Public Trust*. San Francisco: Sierra Club Books.
3. National Institute for Occupational Safety and Health (NIOSH). 1986. *Proposed National Strategy for the Prevention of Leading Work-Related Diseases and Injuries: Severe Occupational Traumatic Injuries*. Cincinnati: NIOSH.
4. National Safety Council. 1998. *Safety + Health* May.
5. Castelli, Jim. 1992. "Regulations Get a Red Light." *Safety + Health* September.
6. AFL-CIO. 1998. *Death on the Job: The Toll of Neglect; A State-by-State Profile of Worker Safety and Health in the United States*. Washington: AFL-CIO.

CHAPTER 2

Our Future at Risk

Karen could not control her excitement. She was going to have a baby. She did not have to say a word to her husband, David. He had seen that expression before and he knew what it meant.

He held her and she let herself relax in the shelter of his arms. "It will be different this time," he said. "I promise."

She nodded but did not answer, her thoughts drifting back to the year before when she had brought her husband the same news. She did not like to think about the past, but the empty nursery across the hall was a constant reminder. As painful as it was to see the unused crib and the brightly colored wallpaper in the room, Karen and David had let the room remain as it was, not as a memorial to their grief but as a testament to their faith that she would once again conceive and this time carry the baby to term.

"I hope so," Karen said, finally.

It didn't take long for the word to get out at the dental office where Karen worked. Even Dr. O'Neil had something to say about it.

"So, my number one dental hygienist is going to be leaving me soon to be a mommy? Is that what I hear?" he said.

"Not really all that soon," she said. "I'll work just as long as I can."

"Don't worry about it. Just take care of yourself," the dentist said. "You're very lucky, you know. Sandy and I have been trying for three years without success."

Lucky? Karen wouldn't call herself that. She had lost her first baby early in her pregnancy and her doctor could not find any reason to explain her miscarriage. She had been so careful—eating the right foods, watching her weight, no smoking, no drinking—but still it had happened. Now she was pregnant once again and worried. If she didn't know what had caused the first miscarriage, how could she be sure it would not happen again?

When she woke suddenly from a sound sleep a few nights later, the excruciating cramps doubling her over in pain, she knew her nightmare had become real. It was happening again.

David bundled her into the car and sped off to the hospital, but Karen knew it was too late. Nothing could save her baby. As the sedative began to take hold, just before she fell asleep, she imagined once again the still-empty nursery.

Even though Karen took all the necessary precautions to ensure that her pregnancy was a healthy one, she lost her baby. What Karen did not know was that both her miscarriages were not caused by anything she had done or failed to do. She lost her babies because of her job.

As a dental hygienist, Karen had been frequently exposed to nitrous oxide, a gas commonly used as an anesthetic in dental offices and in hospital operating rooms. Sometimes called "laughing gas," nitrous oxide has been shown to have serious effects on the reproductive systems of women, and to a lesser extent, men. The reproductive effects of nitrous oxide are very serious: miscarriages (spontaneous abortions), reduced fertility, and neurologic, renal, and liver diseases in children born to mothers exposed to the gas. In a 1992 study by A. S. Rowland and other researchers, published in the *New England Journal of Medicine*, it was discovered that female dental assistants who were exposed to nitrous oxide for five hours or more per week had reduced fertility compared to females who were not exposed to the gas. The exposed assistants had a 59 percent decrease in probability of conception for any given menstrual cycle compared with the unexposed assistants.[1]

Dr. O'Neil, like most dentists using nitrous oxide today, had a scavenging system in use. This equipment is designed to protect the dentist and his assistants from inhaling the gas by collecting it from places in which it may be leaking, most notably gas lines or the patient's mask used to administer the gas. Even with Dr. O'Neil's safety precautions, Karen was exposed to enough nitrous oxide during her three-year employment as his dental hygienist to have suffered two miscarriages. The inability of Dr. O'Neil's wife to conceive may also have been linked to his own exposure to the gas, which may have affected the viability of his sperm.

Health care professionals working in dental offices or hospital operating rooms have believed themselves protected from nitrous oxide because scavenging systems were in use. In the May 25, 1994, *Update*, the National Institute for Occupational Safety and Health (NIOSH) reported that their studies indicated nitrous oxide exposures as high as 12 times the NIOSH recommended limit in some hospital operating rooms and more than 40 times the NIOSH recommended limit in some dental offices, despite the fact that scavenging systems were in use in both settings.

"These devices may have created a false sense of

security in health care workers. Employers must ensure that these systems provide the expected level of protection," said NIOSH Director Dr. Linda Rosenstock. "Health care workers should not have to risk their health to improve the health of others," she stressed.[2]

The Problem

Reproductive effects caused by an unhealthful workplace are not unique to health care workers. These effects are egalitarian and cut across a wide range of occupations, affecting both blue-collar and white-collar workers, unskilled laborers and highly trained professionals, men and women. Certain cancers, infertility, impotence, miscarriages, low birth weight babies, birth defects, congenital mental retardation, and various genetic diseases are all possible reproductive effects of exposures to workplace toxins and poisons.

The disastrous reproductive effects that are caused by some chemicals first attracted public attention in the 1960s when mothers who had taken the prescription drug thalidomide delivered babies with grotesque physical deformities. In the 1970s, as many as 66 percent of the women whose mothers had been given DES (diethylstilbestrol) during their pregnancies developed abnormal sex organ anatomy. Many of these "DES daughters" also developed an unusual tumor known as clear cell vaginal adenocarcinoma.[3] While thalidomide and DES were chemicals that were encountered in the form of prescription drugs and not in the workplace, the incidence of such severe reproductive effects focused attention on all chemicals and created a heightened awareness of their potentially dangerous effects. These cases demonstrated how intimate was the physical bond between mother and developing fetus and pointed out the ease with which the fetus could be damaged without adversely affecting the health of the mother at all.

Reproductive effects, even when very severe, are sometimes difficult to attribute to the workplace. In California's Central Valley a migrant farm worker gave birth to a baby boy who was born without arms and legs. The woman worked in the raisin grape industry and was exposed to a potent assortment of chemicals used as fertilizers and insecticides. As her case was investigated it was discovered that the woman had daily contact with two chemicals used as fungicides in the fields. These two chemicals, captan and benomyl, were found in the dust that covered the woman's clothes and lingered in the dusty air that she breathed while at work. Further, she quenched her thirst on the job by eating grapes which had been sprayed with the chemicals; she also used grape leaves for her personal hygiene after she relieved herself in the fields. The woman sued the chemical manufacturers, claiming that captan and benomyl were responsible for her son's gross deformities. The case was settled out of court.[4]

The Chevron Corporation, which manufactured captan, stated that the chemical had been tested to see whether it could cause birth defects and the results had been negative. However, one expert has charged that the negative findings were misrepresented and that the data showed that capton could cause birth defects in hamsters, rabbits, and mice.[5] While benomyl was not used very widely in the U.S., researchers in Russia found evidence suggesting that the chemical could cause birth defects.

Of the more than 100,000 chemicals in commercial use today, only 1,600 have been tested to see if they cause birth defects (the Organizational Corporation of Economic Development considers 35,000 synthetic chemicals to have adverse health effects in humans). How many of these chemicals are capable of horrible reproductive effects? The fact that the cause of 55 to 70 percent of all birth defects observed in children today remains unknown should be reason enough to study the effects of chemical agents on the developing fetus.

But to fully understand the magnitude of reproductive effects caused by exposures to synthetic chemicals in the workplace is to understand that the problem is much more than just birth defects.

In 1976, a group of men were talking in the locker room at a pesticide production facility of Occidental Petroleum in Lathrop, California. In the casual conversation of these workers, it turned out that many of them, an unusually high number in fact, had been unable to father children. Researchers who investigated this strange problem found that 35 of the 114 men examined had abnormal sperm counts, and even worse, 15 of them could produce no sperm at all. The researchers found that the one commonality among the men most severely affected was their exposure to DBCP (1,2-dibromo-3-chloropropane), a chemical used as a soil sterilant and nematode poison.[6]

As early as 1961, research had shown that DBCP was capable of producing atrophy of the testes, but this knowledge was not incorporated into industrial safety practices or warning sheets. Were it not for their locker-room talk, the workers at Occidental Petroleum would never have known that their inability to father children was caused by a workplace exposure to a dangerous chemical and that the problem was widespread. In 1978, DBCP was banned in California and one year later, all interstate commerce of the chemical was banned, although Shell Oil and Dow Chemical, the major manufacturers of DBCP, continued to export the chemical abroad. In 1983, a jury awarded approximately $5 million to seven workers in their suit against Dow and Shell for their fertility impairment caused by workplace exposures to DBCP.

The Occidental Petroleum example demonstrates how difficult it is to identify workplace hazards as a cause of reproductive effects. Any one of the men involved, taken singly, would not have suspected DBCP to be the culprit behind his fertility impairment. Drugs, alcohol, disease, injury, and a whole litany of other factors could have been the causative agents behind any of the workers' problems. The chances are very good that any physician examining one of the men would not have uncovered DBCP as the problem.

Synthetic chemicals such as PCBs, CFCs (chlorofluorocarbons used in aerosols and sprays), pesticides such as DDT, and many others have saturated our environment to the point where a researcher would be hard-pressed to find any living thing that does not harbor at least a molecule or two of one or more of these toxic substances. With 100,000 such chemicals already on the market worldwide and 1,000 new ones produced each year, we are creating a potent chemical environment whose future health effects are anyone's guess.

A Danish team of researchers, headed by Dr. Niels Skakkebaek, reviewed 61 international studies of semen analysis performed on men since 1938 and published their findings in the September 1992 edition of the *British Medical Journal*. The team discovered that the average male sperm count had dropped 45 percent from 1940 to 1990.[7] It is important to note the years covered by the study, since synthetic chemicals really came into their own during World War II and have been a part of our lives ever since. While some scientists were skeptical of the Danish team's results, at least three other studies performed since then in Belgium, France, and Scotland have confirmed that sperm counts have dropped, most likely as a result of environmental causes.[8] Although these studies were not necessarily linked to workplace exposures to toxic chemicals, it is fair to say that the workplace is a likely site of exposure.

NIOSH has put together a laundry list of chemicals that are used in a variety of workplaces and that have been shown to have potential adverse reproductive effects. The list includes:

Aldrin—spontaneous abortion, premature labor

Arsenic—spontaneous abortion, decreased birth weight, congenital defects, developmental defects

Benzene—spontaneous abortion, low birth weight, menstrual disorders, ovarian atrophy

Cadmium—low birth weight

Carbon disulfide—spontaneous abortion, menstrual disorders, adverse effects on sperm

Chlorinated compounds such as TCE, PCE, and chloroform—eye, ear, and oral cleft anomalies, central nervous system disorders, perinatal deaths, childhood leukemia

Dichloroethylene—congenital heart disease

Dieldrin—spontaneous abortion, premature labor

Hexachlorocyclohexane—spontaneous abortion, premature labor, hormonal imbalance

Lead—impotence, decreased sex drive, sterility, spontaneous abortion, low birth weight, stillbirth, preterm delivery, neurobehavioral deficits, mental retardation, adverse effects on sperm and testes

Mercury—spontaneous abortion, menstrual disturbances, blindness, deafness, mental retardation, delayed development, brain damage

1,2-dibromo-3-chloropropane—adverse effects on sperm, sterility

Polychlorinated biphenyls—low birth weight, preterm

delivery, reduced head circumference, growth deficiencies, neurobehavioral effects

Polycyclic aromatic hydrocarbons (PAHs)—decreased fertility

Trichloroethylene—congenital heart disease.

Remember that this is only a partial list of chemicals with *known* adverse reproductive outcomes; time will tell how many other chemicals currently circulating in our workplaces, or yet to come, will be as dangerous.

How Does It Happen?

How do these chemicals actually cause reproductive effects in humans? Much of it has to do with how they interfere with our body's endocrine system.

The endocrine system is responsible for manufacturing and releasing hormones into the bloodstream. Hormones are chemical messengers that help regulate the proper workings of the body and urge it to begin certain processes when necessary. A variety of organs, known as endocrine glands, produce the hormones that then travel through the blood to affect the workings of other parts of the body. For example, estrogens produced in a woman's ovaries travel to the uterus, where they "tell" the womb to prepare for possible pregnancy. The body's metabolism is directed by hormones from the thyroid while growth hormones that regulate development are manufactured in the brain's pituitary gland. The pituitary is also "control central," the master gland that regulates the activities of all the body's hormones. The endocrine system is extremely complex and relies on a constant communication between hormones and organs for its proper functioning. A disruption of this system at any point can have unexpected, and sometimes disastrous, results in areas of the body far removed from the site of interference.

Research shows that synthetic chemicals in the workplace may interfere with the endocrine system by imitating hormones, blocking hormone receptors, or inhibiting or stimulating hormone production or degradation.[9] For example, a chemical that blocked the effect of testosterone, an important hormone in male sexual development, may result in a male baby born with an undescended testicle or perhaps a low sperm count, an effect that would not show up until much later in life. A chemical that imitates a hormone may trigger some bodily process at a time when it is not needed, perhaps causing unwanted results in metabolism or development. Timing is everything in fetal development as growth processes normally proceed along a precise schedule, regulated by hormones. Depending on when a synthetic chemical interferes with the process, the effects of its action may be demonstrated immediately in the fetus or newborn, or may not be apparent until later in life, or may have no effect at all. For example, thalidomide, taken by a woman very late in her pregnancy, has no adverse effects on the fetus, unlike the deformities that it causes in earlier stages of pregnancy.

For many years it was thought that the placenta—the tissue attached to the wall of the womb that connects to the fetus through the umbilical cord—acted as a sort of shield to protect the developing fetus from any poisons taken in by the mother. That assumption was rocked when the first reports about horrible birth defects caused by thalidomide, taken by pregnant women as a tranquilizer or for nausea, began to surface. Less than a decade later, the high incidence of vaginal cancer in young women whose mothers had taken diethylstilbestrol (DES) during their pregnancies—ironically to prevent miscarriages and to promote bigger, healthier babies—proved conclusively that the placenta was not the impenetrable barrier medical science had thought it was and that, in fact, a fetus was at risk of being adversely affected by chemicals in the mother's bloodstream. Recently, we have been seeing sad examples of this principle at work as babies are being brought into the world addicted to alcohol and narcotics, or infected by the AIDS virus.

What we now know is that pregnant women should be extremely careful about the chemicals they ingest through smoking and drinking, diet, medication, and environmental exposure, including exposures in the workplace.

The synthetic chemicals at use in the workplace have their own special set of problems, however. All workers, male or female, are already harboring some of these chemicals within their body, a result of the ubiquitous nature of these substances in our environment. The workplace may bring more exposures of the same chemical or may bring exposures to new chemicals, which may interact in unpredictable ways with the chemicals already deposited in body fat. This can be a problem for pregnant or postpartum women. Women who breast-feed may pass these chemicals on to their babies through their milk. In the 1950s, nursing infants in Turkey died from a fatal disease called *pembe yara*, caused by nursing mothers who ate hexachlorobenzene-tainted bread, and maternal and nursing infant neurotoxicity was found in Iraq in the 1970s, caused by methylmercury-tainted bread ingested by nursing mothers.[10]

There is a tendency when speaking about reproductive effects to speak about effects to the organs of the reproductive system itself, as if there were no other bodily effects. However, the list in the previous section enumerates other disorders, including congenital heart disease, leukemia, central nervous system disorders, developmental defects, mental retardation, and brain damage, all of which are most likely a result of hormonal interference in the fetus, causing effects removed from the organs of the reproductive system. What this means is that toxic chemicals in the workplace are not only affecting the reproductive ability of our children and grandchildren, but are also producing a whole class of children who may be mentally deficient or otherwise impaired. Taken together, these effects could have devastating consequences for our progeny worldwide.

For an excellent discussion of the effects of synthetic chemicals upon the endocrine system and what that means for our progeny, we recommend *Our Stolen Future* by Colborn, Dumanoski, and Myers.

No One Is Immune

Let's be clear about one thing; you don't need to work in a high-risk occupation to suffer reproductive effects brought about by your workplace. Just because you may not labor in a field enveloped in a cloud of pesticides does not mean that you are free from workplace toxins. They are everywhere, insidious, and ever present.

Nor are adverse reproductive effects a problem only for women, although women are most often the focus of questions about occupational hazards to reproduction. This may reflect a tendency to view birth defects or other adverse pregnancy outcomes only as disorders of reproduction. In addition, as women move into previously all-male jobs, their reproductive health may be a matter of concern, mostly because they may bring a third party—the embryo/fetus—into the equation. Meanwhile, men who have traditionally been in the workplace are assumed to be unaffected, even though little information is available to substantiate this. In fact, as we have seen, there is good reason for further study of occupational hazards to male reproduction.

Let's look at some workplaces that may pose reproductive risks for both women and men.

Karen's case points out how the health of health care workers is often compromised by their work. In hospitals, surgeons, anesthetists, and nurses may all be exposed to nitrous oxide at dangerous levels.

Often there is a perception among hospital workers that some risks are just part of their job and there is little that can be done about them. How nurses handle ribavirin, a drug administered to infants with life-threatening respiratory problems, is a good example. The drug may save an infant's life, but it has also been shown to have adverse reproductive effects in animals, and therefore there is concern that it may have a similar effect in women. Under normal circumstances a nurse will not be unduly exposed to ribavirin since it is given in the form of a mist in an enclosed incubator. However, if the infant should be in medical distress, the nurse will immediately open the incubator, rather than wait a few minutes for administration of the drug to be stopped and for the incubator to be cleared. While this may be the necessary step to take in an emergency, it does result in the nurse's exposure to ribavirin.

Workers in hospital supply services use ethylene oxide in order to sterilize medical equipment and surgical instruments. This gas has been shown to increase the risk of miscarriages.[11] NIOSH also recommends that ethylene oxide be regarded as a potential occupational carcinogen.

Some medical instruments, most notably those used in endoscopic and respiratory procedures, are sterilized in a diluted bath of glutaraldehyde. While glutaraldehyde itself has not yet been shown to have reproductive effects, the chemical is closely related to other aldehydes that have demonstrated such effects.[12] Still, nurses and other health care workers are continually exposed to glutaraldehyde solution.

Even medical workers who repair broken instruments

containing mercury, such as thermometers and sphygmomanometers (blood-pressure-reading instruments), are at risk of suffering reproductive effects. Exposure to mercury has caused menstrual disturbances and miscarriages and has caused children to be born blind, deaf, or mentally retarded, and displaying delayed development and brain damage. Since mercury is used in dental offices in amalgams, dental professionals are also at risk.

No one would consider picking up their laundry at a dry cleaning store to be a very risky task but in their daily work, dry cleaners are continually exposed to solvents such as chloroform and a chemical known as TCE (trichloroethylene). Children born to women who have had excessive exposures to these chemicals have suffered from deformities of the eyes and ears and some have been stricken with disorders of the central nervous system and childhood leukemia. In severe conditions, the child dies shortly after birth.[13]

Workers in other industries in which chloroform is used are also stricken by the same reproductive effects. Some of these industries include the manufacture of refrigerants, plastics, and aerosol propellants. Chloroform is also used as a solvent and in some photographic processing.

We know how dangerous insecticides can be but rarely think about the health of our friendly lawn-service man as he sprays our lawn and we never think about those who actually work in the factories where these poisons are made. Worse, these workers themselves are not giving much thought to their health and that of their future progeny as they go about their daily tasks ignorant of, or at least insufficiently concerned about, the chemicals they are handling.

Chemicals such as arsenic, benzene, aldrin, carbon disulfide, and dieldrin are routinely used as insecticides.

As a group, these chemicals are known to have devastating reproductive effects on both men and women. Farmworkers who use these chemicals are especially at risk. Some of the documented side effects include: miscarriages, premature labor, low birth weight babies, congenital disorders, menstrual disorders, reduced sperm production, and impaired sperm motility.

Workers in other industries that use these chemicals are susceptible to the same type of reproductive effects. As an example, arsenic is used in metallurgy to harden copper, lead, and alloys, and is also used in the smelting of copper ores. It is used in the production of pigments and in the manufacture of some types of glass, and in the form of gallium arsenide is extensively used in the manufacture of semiconductors.

Benzene, another chemical in the group, is found in gasoline and is used in the chemical industry to produce other organic chemicals. Benzene is also used to manufacture detergents, solvents, and paint removers.

When we think of the occupational health problems that may exist for highway workers and road builders, we do not often think of reproductive effects. We probably think first of accidents, but it has been shown that exposures to some hydrocarbons, commonly found in vehicle exhaust emissions and in asphalt, can cause decreased fertility.[14] These same hydrocarbons are also present in coal tar, the smoke from fires, and even tobacco smoke.

Mechanics and auto repair workers are exposed to these hydrocarbons, but they also have many other dangerous chemicals surrounding them in the workplace: benzene, TCE found in degreasing solvents, PCE (perchloroethylene) in solvents and cleaners, lead in storage batteries, and PCBs (polychlorinated biphenyls) in hydraulic fluid. Besides the reproductive effects already noted for benzene and TCE, lead is associated with stillbirths, miscarriages, preterm deliveries, low birth weight babies, impotence, sperm abnormalities, and neurologic disorders in infants. PCBs also cause preterm deliveries and low birth weight babies and may cause reduced head circumference in infants, growth deficiencies, and neurobehavioral effects.

By now, you should understand that surrounding us every day in the workplace there are many chemicals exhibiting severe reproductive effects. There are thousands more about which we do not yet know enough to determine whether or not they are safe. It is likely that, sooner or later, our paths will cross with one or more of them.

Protecting Our Future

How do we protect ourselves and our future, our progeny, from dangerous reproductive effects found in our workplaces? That is not an easy question to answer. Because reproductive effects do not usually occur immediately, their results cannot be seen until it is too late. If a carpenter falls off a ladder and receives a concussion, there is an immediate and undeniable cause-and-effect relationship at work. Reproductive effects, no matter how they are caused, may not appear for several months, or even years, and when they do, it becomes very difficult to link their origins to specific occupational hazards. (Who would have thought that lack of sex drive could be a result of chemical exposures on the job?) Too many other factors can confuse the picture. Diet, general health of the mother, genetic factors, and substance abuse are just some of the other conditions that could result in reproductive effects.

In order to protect yourself, you must become as knowledgeable as possible about the health and safety hazards that you encounter in your workplace. The Hazard Communications Standard that was established by the Occupational Safety and Health Administration (OSHA) requires by law that all employers inform their employees of any and all risks to their safety and health that may be experienced as a result of their job. It is essential to note that even with this standard in place many employers, either through negligence, ignorance, or deliberate noncompliance, fail to educate their employees about workplace hazards. It is essential that you take responsibility for your own well-being in the workplace, especially as new technologies and new chemicals appear, increasing our safety and health risks.

One way you can find out about reproductive effects on your job is to make use of the Material Safety Data Sheets (MSDS) that the employer is obliged to have on file for every product in use at that workplace. This legal requirement is part of the Hazard Communications Standard and protects your right to know about any unsafe materials you may be using, or are exposed to, while on the job. You have access to this information and can request copies for your own use. Read the data carefully, however. OSHA requires certain information to be included in all MSDS but does not regulate the format in which that information is presented. Because of this, it may be difficult to get an accurate appraisal of your risks solely through the data, which is written by the manufacturer.

It would be a good idea for a pregnant woman, or one who is trying to conceive, to give her obstetrician or gynecologist a copy of the MSDS so that the physician may evaluate any reproductive effects that may be listed in the data. This would also be a wise thing to do for any man who may be trying to start a family. The key thing to remember here is that the first trimester of pregnancy is very critical to the overall health of the developing fetus. It is strongly recommended that any woman who may be exposed to chemicals or other health hazards in her workplace consult with her physician about those hazards before conception ever takes place.

Some companies have established fetal protection policies that are designed to protect women from reproductive effects in the workplace. Fetal protection policies generally work by excluding women, a discriminatory practice, rather than by making the workplace safe for them. Under such policies a woman can be denied a particular job or transferred to a less hazardous job. While this action may eliminate any threat to her unborn baby or her ability to conceive, it may be a two-edged sword for the woman involved. If a "safe" job at the same pay rate cannot be found for her, the woman may be placed on disability leave with full benefit coverage throughout her pregnancy, childbirth, and recovery. Not only is the woman denied the opportunity to work but she also becomes a financial burden for the employer. This helps to explain why some companies have declared specific jobs, because of their inherent reproductive risks, to be off-limits to women of childbearing age. Rather than paying for long-term disabilities or facing the possibility of lawsuits being brought against them by women who have suffered reproductive effects caused by their workplace environment, these companies simply avoid the problem by not allowing women to work in dangerous capacities. This type of discrimination ostensibly protects the woman and her offspring, but the net effect is that some doors in the workplace remain closed to women simply because they are women.

Discrimination of this sort has forced some women into making heartbreaking decisions, choosing between a job and economic security or a family. There have been cases in which women have chosen sterilization in order to keep a job that has known adverse reproductive effects and would have resulted in their exclusion if they were capable of becoming pregnant. An example is the chemical company that had a policy of excluding "women of childbearing potential" from workplaces involving lead exposures. Still, under its "general duty" clause, OSHA alleged that the company had adopted a policy that required women workers to be sterilized in order to continue working in one of its lead departments. The company denied that it had encouraged such a drastic step, but it is a measure of the subtle power the company held over its employees' lives that these women would have felt compelled to make such a devastating decision. It is a decision no worker should ever have to make. Defending the OSHA citation, former Assistant Secretary of Labor Eula Bingham said, "No worker must be forced to sacrifice his or her right to conceive children in order to hold a job."[15]

Still, many women continue to voluntarily sign waivers in which they agree to accept the reproductive risks inherent in their workplaces and further agree not to hold the company responsible should those effects occur. One wonders whether these women, and those choosing voluntary sterilization, are being given all the facts in an objective manner and truly understand the long-term effects to which they are exposing themselves.

There are definite steps that a corporation can take to protect its employees from workplace-induced reproductive disorders. These include:

- Identifying known reproductive hazards in the workplace
- Disseminating information about these hazards to any worker who may be affected by them

- Developing control technologies or work practices that would reduce the worker's risk of exposure to these hazards
- Substituting less toxic substances for harmful ones wherever possible
- Establishing a medical surveillance program that would monitor workers exposed to chemicals with known or suspected reproductive effects
- Developing workers' training programs and monitoring their implementation and effectiveness.

A program like this, which is really quite basic, is the first step toward protecting ourselves and our children, but it is not enough. We must try to change the workplace to make it safe for everyone. Somehow, our employers must be made to see that it makes sense, morally, legally, and financially, to provide safer workplace environments than it does to fight against change. Our future depends upon it.

References

1. Rowland, Andrew S. et al. 1992. "Reduced Fertility Among Women Employed as Dental Assistants Exposed to High Levels of Nitrous Oxide." *New England Journal of Medicine* 327:14.
2. Ibid.
3. Colborn, Theo, Dianne Dumanoski and John Peterson Myers. 1996. *Our Stolen Future*. New York: Plume.
4. Lappe, Mark. 1991. *Chemical Deception: The Toxic Threat to Health and the Environment*. San Francisco: Sierra Club Books.
5. Ibid.
6. Mokhiber, Russell. 1989. *Corporate Crime and Violence: Big Business and the Abuse of the Public Trust*. San Francisco: Sierra Club Books.

7. Colborn, Theo, Dianne Dumanoski and John Peterson Myers. 1996. *Our Stolen Future.* New York: Plume.
8. Ibid.
9. National Institute for Occupational Safety and Health (NIOSH). 1994. *Reproductive Hazards in the Workplace Bibliography.* Cincinnati: NIOSH.
10. Fisher, Jeffrey et al. 1997. "Lactational Transfer of Volatile Chemicals in Breast Milk." *American Industrial Hygiene Association Journal* 58:425-431.
11. National Institute for Occupational Safety and Health (NIOSH). 1989. *Ethylene Oxide Sterilizers in Health Care Facilities.* Cincinnati: NIOSH.
12. National Institute for Occupational Safety and Health (NIOSH). 1991. *Carcinogenicity of Acetaldehyde and Malonaldehyde, and Mutagenicity of Related Low-Molecular-Weight Aldehydes.* Cincinnati: NIOSH.
13. Lappe, Mark. 1991. *Chemical Deception: The Toxic Threat to Health and the Environment.* San Francisco: Sierra Club Books.
14. National Institute for Occupational Safety and Health (NIOSH). 1994. *Reproductive Hazards in the Workplace Bibliography.* Cincinnati: NIOSH.
15. LaDou, Joseph. 1981. *Occupational Health Law: A Guide for Industry.* New York: Marcel Dekker, Inc.

CHAPTER 3

The Invisible Killer

He was still about two hundred yards from the pin, but Frank's tee shot was a beauty, straight down the fairway.

"Lucky shot, Frank," one of his golfing buddies joked.

Frank did think he was lucky. It was a beautiful day, he felt terrific, and if his game kept up like this he was going to win a few bucks from his foursome.

Frank was walking to the cart when suddenly he was seized with a pain that doubled him over. His friends rushed to help him where he stood clutching his belly, groaning in agony.

His partners hurried him back to the clubhouse. The pain, as intense as it was, did not last and Frank was feeling better only a few minutes later. He refused his friends' offer to take him to the hospital, laughing off his attack as something he ate that didn't agree with him.

The following day he was back at the plant where he worked, a factory that manufactured rubber gaskets. Twenty-two years on the job had taught him all the shortcuts and he thought he had it pretty easy, certainly better than a lot of other guys his age.

Three days after his aborted golf outing, while he was at the plant, Frank was again seized with pain so severe that he could not continue to work. The employee health nurse at the plant could find no explanation for the attack and sent him home with some aspirin and a recommendation that he see his doctor.

"Frank, quit being so stubborn. You've got to see a doctor," insisted his wife when he suffered yet another attack at home a day later.

"It's nothing, Liz. I'm all right."

"How can you say that? I worry about you, Frank. You're 53 and I can't remember when you last saw a doctor."

"Saturday, on the golf course," he said, but she did not laugh.

He began to take his condition more seriously as the attacks continued and he started to lose weight. It seemed that no matter how much he ate, he couldn't keep the weight on. Reluctantly, he agreed to a complete physical examination.

Frank's doctor noticed some irregularities in his patient's blood work and referred him to a specialist, an oncologist. Time suddenly seemed to fast-forward for Frank as X rays revealed that his liver was grossly enlarged. A liver biopsy determined that he had angiosarcoma, a rare form of liver cancer.

The doctor's prognosis was grim; Frank had little more than six months to live.

It is estimated that there are 17,000 new cases of occupationally induced cancers reported each year.[1] Many more people than that die each year as a result of occupational cancers, but the actual numbers are hard to determine since the cancer usually occurs decades after the exposures that caused the disease process began. Other related factors such as smoking, diet, environment, lifestyle, heredity, and additional disease states can also contribute to an individual's cancer, making it difficult to pinpoint the cause to the workplace.

In Frank's case, it was determined that his angiosarcoma was a direct result of continued exposure to vinyl chloride, a chemical used in the manufacture of rubber. A cancer with such a specific cause-and-effect relationship is known as a "marker" cancer and is relatively uncommon. It is precisely because they are uncommon, yet so specific, that physicians are able to directly link these cancers to workplace conditions. Another classic case of a "marker" cancer involved workers in the watch and clock industry who painted the faces of these instruments with radium to make them luminous. The painting was precise, finely detailed work and the painters would keep a sharp tip on their brushes by inserting them in their mouths and drawing them out, much as a tailor puts a point on a thread. Each time the workers inserted the brushes in their mouths, they ingested some radium. An unusually high rate of bone cancer developed among these workers and their disease was conclusively linked to radium.[2]

Unfortunately for researchers, "marker" cancers are relatively rare. Most occupational cancers are of more common varieties and thus are not generally detectable until long after the initial exposure to a carcinogen began.

Our knowledge of carcinogens in the workplace and the resulting cancers they cause is only in its infancy. Even though Sir Percival Pott, in 1775, first linked cancer of the scrotum among chimney sweeps to their occupational exposures to soot and tar, it was not until the twentieth century that the particular mechanisms of carcinogenesis and the specific carcinogenic components of soot and tar were discovered. We are just now beginning to understand the dangers inherent in some carcinogenic workplace agents. Even as we grapple with this elementary knowledge, new links between cancer and workplace carcinogens are being discovered on a routine basis.

Despite that, the National Cancer Institute allocates only about 1 percent of its annual budget to study cancer caused by workplace carcinogens.

The Problem

The incidence of occupational cancers is one of staggering proportions, even by the most conservative estimates. Data collected in 1972 by the National Institute for Occupational Safety and Health (NIOSH) suggested that 110,000 workers were potentially exposed to the 21 chemicals then regulated by the Occupational Safety and Health Administration (OSHA) as carcinogens.[3] There are many more chemicals in use in the workplace for which OSHA does not yet have regulatory standards but which are also considered carcinogenic. If exposures to these chemicals are included, then the number of workers with potential exposures to occupational carcinogens balloons to at least 3 million and perhaps as high as 9 million. A 1982 article in the *American Journal of Industrial Medicine* stated that as many as 27.5 million workers may have had past exposures to asbestos alone, a known carcinogen that affects the lungs, pleura, and peritoneum.[4]

One of the most difficult questions a worker may ask a safety officer or industrial hygienist is "Will this stuff give me cancer?" A second, more enlightened question is "Will what I do with this stuff cause cancer?" In order to answer these questions, two processes must be employed. The first is to analyze the chemicals in question through scientific studies to determine whether or not they have a carcinogenic effect in humans. The second method is to perform a thorough risk assessment of the situation.

There are several international agencies that have reviewed hundreds of workplace chemicals to determine whether or not they can cause cancer in humans. These agencies include: American Conference of Governmental Industrial Hygienists (ACGIH), International Agency for Research on Cancer (IARC), Deutsche Forshungsgemeinschaft Commission (DFG), Environmental Protection Agency (EPA), National Institute for Occupational Safety and Health (NIOSH), National Toxicology Program (NTP), and Occupational Safety and Health Administration (OSHA). These various agencies use different rating systems, so chemicals may be classified differently depending upon the particular agency. For example, captafol, a fungicide, is listed as "probably carcinogenic to humans" by IARC, "carcinogenic" by NIOSH, and "not classifiable as a human carcinogen" by ACGIH. The differences in these agencies' rating systems points out how difficult it is to accurately link a given chemical to cancer, both because of the long lag time before the cancer can be diagnosed and because of other health conditions that may be present in the affected individual.

All seven agencies classify eleven chemicals as carcinogenic. They are acrylonitrile; arsenic; asbestos; benzene; benzidine; cadmium; bis-chloromethyl ether; chloromethyl methyl ether; 3, 3'-dichlorobenzidine; N,N-dimethylnitrosamine; and formaldehyde. Six of the agencies list an additional twenty-seven substances as carcinogenic. Some of these are: 2-naphthylamine, which causes bladder cancer; chromium and chromates, lung and nasal sinuses cancer; coke oven emissions, lung and kidney cancer; and wood dust, which causes cancer of the nasal cavity.

Identifying chemicals as to their potential to cause cancer is only a small part of what is known as risk assessment. It is important to understand the concept of risk assessment, not only in the case of cancer but for other workplace diseases as well, so we'll take a closer look at the principles involved in risk assessment.

According to *The Occupational Environment—Its Evalua-*

tion and Control, published by the American Industrial Hygiene Association, risk assessment is defined as "the process of determining, either quantitatively or qualitatively, the probability and magnitude of an undesired event and estimating the cost to human society or the environment in terms of morbidity, mortality, or economic impact."[5] It should be noted that risk assessment is not used exclusively to assess the risk of contracting a workplace-induced cancer, but is used to assess the threat of any workplace disease or injury. In the workplace, risk assessment is based upon four parameters: hazard identification, dose response assessment, exposure assessment, and risk characterization.

Let's examine these parameters one at a time.

- **Hazard identification**—As explained above, hazard identification seeks to determine which workplace chemicals or conditions can pose a threat to workers' health. In the case of cancer, chemicals are usually the recognized hazard, but this is not always true for other workplace diseases. Carpal tunnel syndrome, for example, is the result not of a chemical hazard but of a repetitive motion, and some skin cancers are caused by ultraviolet radiation.
- **Dose response assessment**—This term really refers to the toxicity of a chemical. The assessment tries to discover at what dosage a chemical becomes dangerous to human health. While both animal and human studies are used in a dose response assessment, the ideal assessment would be based upon human studies, since there are substantial biochemical, structural, and behavioral differences between humans and animals. Mathematical extrapolations may be made from animal studies to provide an equivalent dosage for humans.
- **Exposure assessment**—The exposure assessment is determined by analyzing the workplace environment,

the workers, and the interactions between the two. In simple terms, this analysis examines the workplace to see how likely it is a worker would be exposed to a dangerous chemical, how often, and how long. It also takes into consideration the worker himself and decides how factors such as age, sex, and overall health may affect his risk of exposure.

- **Risk characterization**—In this final step in the risk assessment process, information from the first three steps are collated, evaluated, and integrated to develop a risk estimate. The goal here is to develop an accurate appraisal of the potential health risks faced by workers who are exposed to the work practices, chemicals, or energies in question.

The risk assessment process is a fairly new tool in occupational safety and health but one that is generally receiving widespread support among professionals in the field. A 1997 NIOSH position paper said that the agency "supports the use of human risk assessment techniques in regulatory decision making, the making of public health policy and in the allocation of government resources to environmental issues."[6]

Still, there are some problems with the risk assessment process caused by the specific methods various agencies use to arrive at a risk estimate. EPA, as an example, calculates what is known as a "plausible conservative" estimate, based on hypothetical numbers and possible exposure scenarios. The agency arrives at this estimate by reviewing animal and human studies (although there are very few of the latter available) and then adding conservative safety margins at various points to account for any plausible risk. "Plausible" does not mean likely to EPA; it means that a risk could occur, even though the odds are against it. The agency's risk estimates, therefore, may be grossly overstated. Betty Anderson, former head of EPA's Carcinogen Assessment Group, has said that the assumptions EPA uses regarding toxicology may overstate the risks by anywhere from 16 times to 10,000-fold.[7]

At a congressional hearing on hazardous waste sites, Thomas Grumbly, Assistant Secretary for Environmental Restoration and Waste Management for the Department of Energy, said:

> EPA contractors come in, turn the crank, use a lot of assumptions that tend to cascade conservative assumption upon conservative assumption, and then hit a particular hazardous waste site with . . . an estimated risk that simply doesn't bear any relationship to what anybody who is knowledgeable actually thinks is a real risk at the site.[8]

But does this mean that a "plausible conservative" assumption is wrong? Politicians, lawyers, and economists who curry favor with corporate America would say yes, such assumptions if enacted into law would require corporations to pay millions of dollars to enact safety measures to protect perhaps that one-in-a-million person who may be at risk. The risk simply does not justify the cost, these naysayers would say. They would point to past notable exaggerations, such as the ideas that saccharin and unleaded gasoline caused cancer—erroneous conclusions that were based on animal studies presumed to be good indicators of how humans would react—and use them as examples of science run amok at the expense of the American economy.

But at least as often the "plausible conservative" assumption proves reasonable. For example, animal studies showed that, 1,3-butadiene, a toxic gas released in the production of rubber, could increase cancer risk to about 8 in 1,000. As a result of these studies, OSHA proposed lowering its permissible exposure limit (PEL) for the chemical from 1,000 ppm (parts per million) to 2 ppm. As expected, the opposition said that the results in mice did not translate to humans and that further regulation of the chemical was unnecessary.

Luckily for thousands of workers, the rubber industry itself conducted human epidemiology studies that confirmed the original animal data. In 1996, the rubber industry and labor unions together asked OSHA to issue a regulation that reduced 1,3-butadiene allowable exposures to no more than 1 ppm, twice as stringent as OSHA's initial proposal.[9] OSHA estimates that about 9,700 workers at 255 facilities are exposed to 1,3-butadiene; the new standard is expected to prevent at least 79 cancer deaths over a 45-year working lifetime.

While EPA is more likely to use a "plausible conservative" approach in formulating a risk estimate, OSHA relies on more realistic numbers and concerns in terms of worker exposures. OSHA is frequently taken to task on the economic front, where businesses often contest the cost of implementing regulations proposed by the agency. It is ironic that OSHA is criticized for overestimating risk estimates while economists and business leaders avoid criticism for their equally inflated estimates of regulatory costs.

In the face of a proposed regulation, economists will determine the cost of implementing it; that figure is often debatable since it reflects only the immediate regulatory cost and overlooks long-term cost analysis. One reason for overestimated costs is the fact that the estimates are often generated by corporate engineers, a group with an obvious allegiance to the corporation's profitability. Also, regulatory costs are overestimated because the control technology that will need to be implemented is most likely not yet available on a large scale, which would reduce its cost.

Despite the dire cost predictions of the economists, OSHA has been fairly accurate in determining regulatory costs. A 1995 report from the Office of Technology Assessment reviewed the costs of seven major regulatory programs mandated by OSHA over the previous fifteen years. The report found that in no case did the regulatory cost exceed the agency's predictions and in five of the cases the costs were lower than predicted.[10]

When estimating regulatory costs, economists fail to include the economic *benefits* that may occur as a result of new regulations. In addition, workers' compensation claims would drop as safety risks are reduced, thereby increasing corporate profits. Also, there will be companies that will benefit from the development and manufacturing of new control equipment and pollution reduction. Citing the high cost to the American economy of regulatory costs is meaningless without also reporting the concomitant economic benefits.

It is important to keep the corporate politicians and their hirelings out of the risk assessment process. Risk estimates need to be made on objective, sound data and not on rhetoric, anecdotes, or flawed studies. Without sound data, no risk estimates can be considered reliable. There is ongoing legislation in Congress designed to help create a reasonable risk assessment policy. Some researchers and industrial hygienists are pushing for the formation of a publicly accessible national data base from which risk assessment and risk management policies can be developed. Workers can best help in this effort by keeping themselves informed of their elected officials' actions relative to risk assessment and by making their opinions known to them.

Cancer at Work

Don't be misled by the fact that seven international agencies agreed that only eleven chemicals cause cancer in humans. When it comes to determining the exact number of workplace carcinogens, the jury is still out. In all likelihood, that number will never be determined. The sheer quantity of different chemicals currently used in the workplace, along with the increasing number of new chemicals developed for new technologies, make the task of identifying every carcinogen impossible. Complicating the problem is that even after researchers discover the carcinogenic potential of a chemical, it may react in a different and surprising manner in combination with other chemicals; sometimes a seemingly innocuous chemical may enhance carcinogenesis. All this means that we just don't know enough yet about carcinogens in the workplace and that workers need to be cognizant of that fact and not simply assume that their workplace is free of a cancer risk.

There are several workplaces in which the risk of cancer is well documented.

Many manufacturing industries, from large automobile manufacturers to small metalworking shops, use metalworking fluids during the machining of metal parts to cool, clean, and lubricate tools and workpieces. Petroleum-based mineral oils are used either alone or as emulsions of oil in water in machining and grinding operations in order to extend tool life, improve the finish on the workpiece, cool and wash away swarf (removed metal shavings), reduce power and force necessary for the cut, and prevent corrosion. At excessive levels these oils may pose a health risk.

These metalworking fluids, also called cutting oils, are generally applied through flooding, a process that delivers a continuous stream of fluid to the tool and the workpiece. Workers in metalworking industries are continually subjected to a spray of cutter oil from the tool while working in a mist of oil produced by condensation of the oil in the high-temperature cutting zone. It is estimated that more than 1 million workers are exposed to cutting oils.[11]

These oils have been associated with acute inflammation of the lungs and with asthma, but their greatest health risk seems to be their role as workplace carcinogens. Skin cancer, a variety of digestive system cancers, including cancer of the large intestine and stomach, and cancer of the rectum, larynx, and prostate have all been linked in varying degrees to exposures to cutting oils.[12]

There are several methods of helping to reduce a worker's exposure to metalworking oils. Substituting water-based coolants for oil-based coolants is one way, although this can't always be done since some manufacturing processes require oil. Air-filtering equipment designed to prevent oil droplets from returning into the factory air is an effective means of reducing exposures, as long as the filters are changed often enough to keep them working properly. Enclosing the machine in a booth also helps to reduce widespread dispersion of the oils, especially if the enclosure is state of the art and is part of the original equipment, as compared to an enclosure that is built afterward. In many processes it may also be possible to reduce the pressure and volume of the cutting oils, or to apply it only when the tool interfaces with the workpiece rather than continually, or to add mist suppressants to the oils to reduce spray. Considering how many workers may be at risk of contracting cancer from exposures to cutting oils, any of these preventive measures are well worth the try.

Construction, furniture refinishing, flexible polyurethane foam manufacturing, leather finishing, aerosol packaging, anesthetic making, paint and stain remover manufacturing, flavoring making, fat extracting, fumigating, and cold degreasing and cold cleaning operations are all examples of industries that rely heavily on methylene chloride for their various processes. This liquid, a widely used solvent, may cause a dry, scaly skin inflammation and even skin burns with prolonged contact. More important, the chemical has been linked to heart disease and cancer.[13]

Cadmium is a bluish-white metal that is high corrosion resistant and is used as a protective coating for iron, steel, and copper as well as for welding electrodes and solders. It is used as an amalgam in dentistry, in electroplating, and in the manufacture of nickel-cadmium batteries, fluorescent lights, semiconductors, photocells, and jewelry. Some cadmium compounds can be found in fungicides, insecticides, pigments, paints, and glass. When the metal form of cadmium is converted into fumes or dust as a result of various manufacturing processes, workers in any of these industries are put at risk.

Exposure to cadmium has been shown to have toxic effects in the kidneys and liver and the metal is a suspected human carcinogen resulting in lung and prostate cancer. Three specific occupations that seem to have an increased risk of contracting cancer through cadmium exposure are battery makers, electroplaters, and welders.

Chromium and chromium compounds are used in similar manufacturing processes as cadmium. Electroplaters, glass workers, lithographers, metalworkers, photoengravers, textile workers, and welders are some of the occupations that are routinely exposed to chromium. Chromium can enter the body either through inhalation or absorption through the skin. Chromium can cause dermatitis, including irritation of the eyes and nasal passages. Research suggests that chromium, in certain forms, is a suspected carcinogen in cancer of the lung, larynx, and nasal cavity. In 1993, after reviewing studies involving welders, the International Institute of Welding/Commission VIII concluded, "On the balance of the evidence from these studies, welders as a group have a slightly greater risk of developing lung cancer than the general population. . . ."[14]

But it's not only exposures to unpronounceable, exotic chemicals that may cause cancer. There are many more common substances in the workplace, everything from oils and soot to police radar guns and pharmaceuticals, that may be carcinogenic.

Firefighters have obvious health risks associated with injury and accidents on the job, but there are also other, less obvious workplace threats to their health. Firemen are not nicknamed "smoke eaters" for nothing, and the smoke they are exposed to as part of their job can be responsible for ailments as minor as dizziness, headache, nausea, and irritation of the eyes and respiratory tract or as serious as a reduction in lung function, pulmonary edema, and lung cancer.

It is soot, fine particulate matter in smoke—especially the smoke from the combustion of oil products like diesel fuel—that is linked to lung cancer. Soot is loaded with chemicals called polycyclic aromatic hydrocarbons, and research has shown that at least eleven of these are carcinogenic to animals and probably to humans as well. Since polycyclic aromatic hydrocarbons can penetrate through the skin, firefighters have an increased risk of exposures to them through both inhalation and percutaneous absorption.

A study conducted by the Department of Occupational Health, Royal Netherlands Navy, was designed to determine the degree of exposure to polycyclic aromatic hydrocarbons experienced by instructors at the Royal

Netherlands Navy fire-fighting school. Trainees at the school are taught how to fight fires, mainly from heating oil, both outside and in a confined space. The study showed that the instructors had a significant increase in the uptake of polycyclic aromatic hydrocarbons over a control group that was not involved in the training exercises (the amount of chemical taken up was determined through urinalysis). Results were even higher for instructors who spent more time in the confined-space training area. The high exposures to polycyclic aromatic hydrocarbons occurred despite the fact that instructors wore respirators while conducting the exercises; instructors also discovered a layer of soot on their naked skin beneath their waterproof clothing, hinting at possible absorption of polycyclic aromatic hydrocarbons through the skin.[15]

Since the Russians first began studying it in the 1960s, there has been increasing interest in researching the link between cancer (generally brain cancer or leukemia) and electromagnetic radiation. This type of radiation, also called non-ionizing radiation, is an ubiquitous part of twentieth-century life, found in such items as microwaves; clock radios; personal computers; televisions; antennas; radar devices; television, radio, and cellular phone broadcast towers; trains; and in the medical field, diathermy machines and electrosurgical units.

There is some evidence to warrant more study into the health effects of electromagnetic radiation, especially in regard to cancer; preliminary studies of rail workers conducted in Japan and Europe appear to indicate an increased risk for brain cancer and leukemia.[16] In 1993, the *American Journal of Industrial Medicine* published a study that showed an increase in testicular cancer among Washington State policemen using handheld radar guns. A study in Great Britain reported statistically significant results for leukemia, skin cancer, and bladder cancer among residents living within ten kilometers of a radio and TV tower. A 1996 study of Polish military personnel exposed to radio frequency magnetism found an increased incidence of cancers of the alimentary canal, brain, and lymphatic system, while in that same year a study of U.S. Air Force personnel with radio frequency exposures, published in the *American Journal of Epidemiology*, showed a statistically significant increase in brain cancer.

At this time, the link between cancer and electromagnetic radiation is not conclusively established. There are a few reasons why this is so. One is that no clear-cut dose-response effect has yet been proven, relative to electromagnetic radiation. While it seems that workers in close proximity to magnetic fields may incur a greater health risk than workers farther away, that theory has not been confirmed. Also, there is still an absence of information on how much exposure workers receive and for how long. Compounding these problems is the difficulty in screening out other forms of electromagnetic radiation in order to find out what workplace exposures exist. There is no doubt, however, that as electromagnetic radiation continues to play an ever-increasing role in our daily lives, researchers will pay more attention to the possible health risks it may entail.

It is ironic that the last group of workers to be discussed, health care workers dedicated to fighting cancer, may themselves be at risk of contracting the disease as a result of workplace exposures. Antineoplastic drugs are pharmaceuticals that are used in chemotherapy to attack rapidly growing cells in the body, such as tumors, and destroy them. Three typical antineoplastic drugs are Adriamycin, cisplatin, and cyclophosphamide. The problem with antineoplastic drugs is that they are unable to recognize healthy cells from unhealthy ones so they will have unwanted effects on various tissues and organs in the human body. For cancer patients, that trade-off is acceptable; they are willing to endure those effects as long as the drugs work on their malignant tumors. For healthy doctors, nurses, and pharmacists who have to work with these dangerous drugs, the trade-off is unacceptable: all side effects and no benefits.

In addition to their possible carcinogenic effects, antineoplastic drugs have other adverse effects, which include irregular menstrual periods and spontaneous abortion, testicular function suppression, hair loss, decreased white blood cells, and liver damage.

Health care workers are exposed to antineoplastic drugs through skin contact as they administer the drugs, although the drugs may also be inhaled, especially in the pharmacy where they are prepared. Nurses and physicians may come into contact with these drugs through aerosolization when the syringe is primed, injected, or removed; through broken or leaking syringes; spills; accidental needle sticks; or improper disposal of used syringes. Since these drugs are excreted from the body in a toxic state, any contact with the patient's excreta may be a source of contamination.

It's Your Life

As we have seen, workplace-induced cancer cuts across many workplaces and may be caused by any number of carcinogenic agents. Cancer is a particularly dangerous workplace disease because it doesn't manifest itself until many years after exposure. Thousands of seemingly healthy workers are already harboring carcinogenic agents that will, at some time in their lives, become full-blown cancers.

So, how can you protect yourself from workplace cancers?

Knowledge is power, and knowing everything you can about the substances you work with every day will help you understand the risks you may be taking. If there are Material Safety Data Sheets available for these substances, read them. But remember that a little knowledge can be dangerous. The information in a Material Safety Data Sheet will tell you what chemicals you are exposed to and in what proportions, and will list noted health effects of those chemicals, but it will not tell you how great of a health risk you are taking by using them. Your true risk factor will be determined by how those chemicals are used. As an example, if you smoke two packs of cigarettes every day, you probably have a high risk of contracting lung cancer. However, if you hold an unopened pack of cigarettes in your hand every day, you run no risk of contracting lung cancer caused by tobacco smoke. It's all in how the carcinogen—in this case, tobacco—is used. Also, Material Safety Data Sheets are written by manufacturers of the chemicals, in their own style, and may be misleading. Just because one manufacturer says "DANGER" while another says "danger" does not necessarily mean that the first is more dangerous than the second.

Remember the saccharin scare and keep in mind that studies performed upon bacteria or animals may not yield the same results in humans. A substance that is *mutagenic*—that is, able to cause mutations in cells—in bacteria or animals may not necessarily be mutagenic in humans. Still, considering the vast unknown of cancer prediction, is it wise to ignore mutagenicity in lower life-forms if there is the possibility that those same or similar mutations may hold true for higher life-forms? Until human studies can yield conclusive results, are you willing to gamble that a couple of bugs who go belly-up in a petri dish have no implications for your future health?

If you're beginning to think that we really just don't know enough about workplace cancer to accurately predict who will contract the disease and how they will contract it, you are right. Epidemiology, the medical science that seeks to discover and understand the interrelationships of the host, agent, and environment in causing disease, holds the key to understanding workplace-induced cancer, but much more work needs to be done in this area.

Surveillance programs offer some help in understanding the epidemiology of workplace cancer and are a necessary first step in protecting workers from the disease. These programs have nothing to do with hidden cameras and industrial spying but everything to do with a thorough safety and medical analysis of the workplace and its health hazards. An exposure surveillance program seeks to characterize physical and chemical agents in the workplace in order to determine how many workers have been exposed, to what extent, and for how long. Medical surveillance programs identify and manage individual cases of illness by the early recognition of latent diseases and by providing health promotion activities.

Such activities would include regular medical exams, possibly with X rays, blood work, and urinalysis. These will help medical staff to diagnose disease and formulate a medical treatment plan.

In exposure surveillance, workers and the workplace are monitored to determine the workers' exposure levels of a given chemical. Various types of industrial hygiene equipment are used to take air samples in the workplace, and in close proximity to the worker, to ascertain this data. Exposures are monitored over time and at routine work hours as well as during special tasks or maintenance. If it is found that some workers have been exposed to potentially harmful levels of the chemical, these workers may then be followed over time to investigate the occurrence of illness.

Data generated in a surveillance program can help the corporation in making decisions that will ensure the health of its workers. As an example, if a chemical used in the workplace is identified as a health hazard, the corporation's safety officer can substitute a nontoxic chemical in its place. If there is no such substitute, the safety officer can try to devise ways to reduce exposures to the chemical, either through new work practices, protective clothing, or control technology such as improved ventilation in the workplace. The same data will inform the safety officer of a particular problem and allow him to research and implement corrective measures.

Sound industrial hygiene principles list, in order of importance, the corrective actions a corporation can take to create a more healthful workplace:

- **Substitution**—replacing the chemical in question with a safer one, or eliminating the offending chemical entirely
- **Engineering controls**—implementing control technology such as ventilation, isolation rooms, better tool design, etc., in order to reduce exposures to the chemical
- **Work practice changes**—changing specific tasks or duties in order to reduce exposures, such as cutting oil being sprayed only when necessary instead of continuously
- **Administrative controls**—reassigning workers to less hazardous jobs or locations, scheduling potentially hazardous tasks at times when less people are in the area
- **Protective clothing**—such as respirators or gloves.

In all likelihood, you probably have little to do with implementing or conducting your company's surveillance program. However, if you have determined your job to be one in which you have some potential risk of contracting a workplace-induced cancer, you should know about the program and whether or not you should be included in it.

Many of the OSHA standards for hazardous chemicals contain requirements for medical surveillance for exposed workers. This means that corporations are required to provide medical exams at no cost to employees exposed to the chemical in question. These exams are usually provided by the company's medical staff, or more likely, by the company's health care provider.

Perhaps more than any other workplace disease, cancer prevention requires you to learn everything you possibly can about your workplace, the substances you use or have contact with, and how your employer is handling the cancer risk. It's a lot of work, but it's worth it. It is your life, after all.

References

1. National Institute for Occupational Safety and Health (NIOSH). 1986. *Proposed National Strategies for the Prevention of Leading Work-Related Diseases and Injuries: Occupational Cancers*. Cincinnati: NIOSH.
2. Ibid.
3. Ibid.
4. Ibid.
5. DiNardi, Salvatore R., ed. 1997. *The Occupational Environment: Its Evaluation and Control*. Fairfax: American Industrial Hygiene Association.
6. American Industrial Hygiene Association (AIHA). 1998. *The Synergist* 9:1.
7. Kenkeremath, Nandan. 1996. "Restoring Reason to Regulation: Applying Scientific Assessment and Cost-Benefit Analysis to Environmental Law." *AIHA Journal* 57:9.
8. Ibid.
9. Finkel, Adam M. 1996. "Myths, Chicanery, and Blundering on the Risk Assessment Front." *AIHA Journal* 57:9.

10. Ibid.
11. Raynor, Peter C., Steven Cooper and David Leith. 1996. "Evaporation of Polydisperse Multicomponent Oil Droplets." *AIHA Journal* 57:12.
12. Ibid.
13. American Conference of Governmental Industrial Hygienists. 1997. *ACGIH Today!* 5:4.
14. American Industrial Hygiene Association (AIHA). 1998. *AIHA Journal* 59:1.
15. Feunekes, F.D.J.R. et al. 1997. "Uptake of Polycyclic Aromatic Hydrocarbons Among Trainers in a Fire-Fighting Training Facility." *AIHA Journal* 58:1.
16. Wenzl, Thurman B. 1997. "Estimating Magnetic Field Exposures of Rail Maintenance Workers." *AIHA Journal* 58:9.

CHAPTER 4

A Fatal Breath

Hector was breathing heavily as he carried the groceries up the stairs to his second-floor apartment. He was sweating—it was a hot July day in the city, after all—but he was surprised to be so out of breath. Could it be his asthma was acting up again, even though it had been 15 years since he last had any difficulty breathing?

He had been working at a muffler and brake shop then, repairing automobile brakes. After a few months on the job he started wheezing and often found himself short of breath. He made a visit to the VA hospital clinic, where he was diagnosed as having asthma. The doctor had prescribed some medication and had given him one of those little pump things that blasted medicine into his lungs.

He set the groceries on the table and tried to take a deep breath but couldn't; his breath was coming in short, raspy gulps instead. His wife, Inez, wasn't home yet and he found himself suddenly worrying about how he would get to the hospital if he needed to. Ridiculous! What was he thinking? He was only 43 years old and strong as his sons; he would be fine.

Hector struggled to throw open the kitchen window and sat heavily in a chair nearby, drinking in the thick cloud that passed for air in the city. After a few minutes, he was breathing normally, and by the time Inez came home from work he was himself again.

He thought he was fine, especially when the temperature soared into the 90s and his breathing was not affected. But then, on a cooler evening a week later, while watching television, his breath suddenly cut out on him. It was as if someone had punched him in the gut and forced all the air out. He felt as though he were suffocating. Inez was terrified and could offer little help. Just when he thought he would pass out, his breathing eased and he slumped in his chair, drained.

The next day Hector went to the clinic, describing his suffering in detail to the doctor. Chest X rays were ordered for the following week. The doctor reviewed the X rays with his patient and pointed out several nodules and lesions in Hector's lungs. That physical evidence, combined with Hector's medical history, left only one diagnosis: asbestosis, a lung disease caused by inhaling asbestos fibers—in Hector's case, fibers inhaled from his many years at the brake shop.

Had the diagnosis been made much earlier, Hector would have had a chance to beat what was now a fatal disease.

Each year millions of workers inhale potentially toxic substances that result in respiratory diseases of varying severity. There are so many of these substances in the workplace that it is difficult to get an accurate number of just how many workers are affected; it is estimated that 2.5 million workers each year are potentially exposed to asbestos alone.

Like many occupational cancers, early recognition of some occupational lung diseases is difficult because the latent period for such diseases may be as long as 15 or even 30 years. This was the case with Hector. By the time his lung disease was diagnosed, it was much too late to do anything about it. In addition, other health factors, such as cigarette smoking, can contribute significantly to the disease process and can mask the link between the disease and workplace exposures to toxic substances.

The Problem

It's relatively easy to become exposed to toxic substances in the workplace—just breathe. There is a wide range of occupational respiratory health problems, some relatively minor, others more severe, even fatal. At one end of the spectrum are simple respiratory irritations such as rhinitis, an inflammation of the sinuses that results in allergylike symptoms such as sneezing, a runny nose, or watery eyes. More severe health problems include asthma and hypersensitivity pneumonitis, an inflammation of the lungs in persons who are particularly sensitive to certain substances. At the far end of the spectrum are generally fatal respiratory diseases such as silicosis, asbestosis, pulmonary edema, and lung cancer.

Silicosis and asbestosis are fibrotic diseases of the lungs; that is, they are characterized by the inhalation and deposition in the lungs of either silica dust or asbestos fibers. These inorganic dusts in the lungs create lesions and nodules that accumulate and eventually grow to a size at which they cut off blood vessels and airways in the lungs, putting a strain on the heart. Ultimately, this could result in heart failure. As if silicosis weren't enough, the International Agency for Cancer Research recently listed silica as a "group 1 carcinogen," which means that silica has been shown to be "a definite cause of cancer in humans."[1]

What is usually regarded as America's worst workplace catastrophe occurred as a result of exposure to silica dust. In 1937, silicosis killed 476 workers constructing the Gauley Bridge in West Virginia, with another 1,500 workers eventually disabled by the disease.

Frances Perkins, the first U.S. Secretary of Labor, was

so incensed by the tragedy that she put special emphasis on trying to eliminate silicosis in the workplace.

"Our job is one of applying techniques and principles to every known silica dust hazard in American industry," she said shortly after the disaster. "We know the methods of control—let us put them into practice."[2]

Despite her plea more than 60 years ago, the threat of silicosis remains high. According to NIOSH, there are 59,000 new cases of silicosis each year and 250 people annually die from the disease. The agency estimates that more than 1 million workers are still exposed to silica dust.[3]

The Occupational Safety and Health Administration (OSHA), the National Institute for Occupational Safety and Health (NIOSH), and the Mine Safety and Health Administration (MSHA) have banded together in a national campaign to eradicate silicosis from the workplace, under the banner "It's Not Just Dust." In 1997, these agencies, along with the American Lung Association, held a national conference in Washington, D.C., to raise awareness of the human and economic costs of silicosis and to discuss methods to battle the disease. At that conference, NIOSH Director Dr. Linda Rosenstock said that NIOSH's recommended exposure level to silica was equivalent to no more than a teaspoon of dust in a football field, a level of exposure that is grossly exceeded in almost any workplace where silica is present.[4]

Which workers are at risk of developing silicosis? Since silica is commonly found in quartz and quartz is found in nearly all mineral deposits and in common rocks such as granite and sandstone, anyone who comes in contact with the dust from rocks or during the course of his workday probably has at least some potential exposure to silica. This would include quarrymen, coal and metal miners, excavators, road builders, sandblasters, and foundry workers, to name a few. Since sand is also used in a variety of industries, such as the glass and pottery industry, and is also used in the production of cement, mortar, bricks, and abrasives, workers in these industries are at risk as well. The same could also be said for workers in soap, paint, and porcelain manufacturing industries since silica flour (silica in a finely pulverized form) is used in these processes.

What About Asbestosis?

Approximately 2.5 million workers are currently exposed to asbestos in the U.S. workplace.[5] However, because of the long latency period required before the disease becomes apparent, former asbestos workers must also be considered at risk, boosting the total number at risk significantly.

While there have been reports of deaths caused by asbestosis as early as the turn of the century, it wasn't until 1928 that the first epidemiologic study regarding the disease was conducted. In Great Britain, the Ministry of Labour studied 363 asbestos workers who were employed in the production of asbestos textiles and discovered a prevalence of pulmonary fibrosis in 80 percent of the workers with 20 years' or more experience on the job.[6] A 1936 study of 100 workers who were dismissed from North Carolina asbestos plants for medical reasons showed that 55 percent of them had moderate to advanced asbestosis; when more than half of a company's workforce comes down with the same disease, that company has a serious problem.

Asbestos is found in a variety of products, including flooring and roofing products; packing and gaskets; thermal and electrical insulation; friction products such as automobile brake linings, coatings, and compounds; textiles; plastics; paper; and asbestos cement sheets and pipe. The largest number of workers exposed to asbestos are involved in the manufacture of these products in such industries as construction, automobile servicing and repair, and shipbuilding.

Workers, as well as the general public, are often exposed to asbestos when repairs or renovations are performed on old buildings that contain asbestos or when the substance is improperly removed from an existing site. Partly fueled by the asbestos industry's initial reluctance to admit to the dangers of asbestos, and spurred on by congressional efforts to address the problem of asbestos in schools, a "fiber phobia" in this country has spawned a $3.9 billion asbestos-removal industry. In the 1980s, with so much money to be made, new asbestos-removal companies with inexperienced and poorly trained workers were springing up overnight.

Even when performed properly, asbestos removal involves disturbing asbestos located in floor tiles, ceiling panels, and insulation and can result in higher asbestos levels than before the removal process began. This was found to be true in a two-year study of a Colorado school in which asbestos was being removed. Asbestos levels were significantly higher after removal, and it was established it would take four years for the levels to recede to where they were before removal.[7]

In 1998, OSHA proposed fines totaling almost $1 million against Interstate Brands Corporation, the manufacturer of Twinkies and other bakery snacks, when three employees were assigned to remove thermal insulation from one of the plant's boilers. OSHA alleged that the insulation contained 75 percent asbestos, but the workers were not informed of that fact.[8] The case is still in litigation.

That same year, OSHA cited the John A. Bellavia construction company of Sunrise, Florida, with several violations because of the company's use of untrained workers to remove asbestos and its failure to provide protection for those workers and to maintain a regulated area for the asbestos removal. The agency proposed fines totaling $100,800, and the company has recently reached agreement with OSHA to pay $25,000 in fines.[9]

"Exposure to asbestos can cause serious illnesses such as lung cancer and asbestosis," said Secretary of Labor Alexis M. Herman. "Workers who handle asbestos must be properly trained in its removal. There is no excuse for an employer to expose workers needlessly to such dangers."[10]

Since the public has become more knowledgeable about the dangers of asbestos, many products that were formerly made from the substance are now asbestos-free.

Coal dust is another inorganic dust that has well-documented respiratory effects. Coal miners' pneumoconiosis, the notorious "black lung," has been a fatal disease for thousands of coal miners around the world. A 1968 explosion at Consolidated Coal Mine No. 9 in Farmington, West Virginia, in which 78 miners were asphyxiated, focused national attention on safety and health issues in the mining industry generally and helped to bring to the public's attention the high incidence of "black lung."

Lorin Kerr, director of occupational safety and health for the United Mine Workers of America (UMWA), said, "At work, coal miners are covered with dust. It's in their hair, their clothes and their skin. It gets between their teeth and they swallow it. They suck so much of it into their lungs that until they die they never stop spitting up coal dust. Some cough so hard, they wonder if they have any lungs left. Gradually, the miners notice they are getting short of breath when they walk up hills. On the job they must stop work to catch their breath. Finally, just walking across the room at home is an effort."[11]

As a result of the Consolidated Coal explosion, new safety laws were quickly enacted to protect workers in the mining industry. Lower dust standards enacted in both the U.S. and U.K.—a country that was publicly battling "black lung" at least 30 years before the U.S. identified the problem—have shown that prevention of the disease is a realistic goal. Recent data also indicates that if a worker is detected with the disease at an early enough stage, moving him to a work area with less dust can still prevent the disease from becoming seriously disabling.[12]

In addition to the inorganic dusts, workers in many occupations are exposed to organic dusts that may result in various respiratory diseases. Dusts from cotton, flax, hemp, coffee, and animal hair are common culprits. A somewhat macabre, but interesting example of organic dust that can cause health problems is human bone ash generated in crematoriums. In a study of Manitoba, Canada, crematorium workers, it was found that human bone ash was stirred up during the sorting process when the remains were sifted and metal objects, such as hip and knee replacements and hardware from the coffin, were removed. It was recommended that, because of the unknown medical condition of the deceased, workers should wear a NIOSH-approved, half-face respirator as they worked.[13]

Not Just Dust

Don't think that you can breathe easy just because you don't work with silica or asbestos. When it comes to respiratory diseases in the workplace, there are many more dangerous agents out there besides dust. There are gases and fumes such as ammonia, carbon dioxide, carbon monoxide, chlorine, hydrogen sulfide, mercury, methane, nitrogen, ozone, phosgene, and sulfur dioxide. There are airborne troublemakers, including thermophilic actinomycetes—bacteria that can be found in moldy compost, moldy sugarcane, and contaminated forced air systems. There are fungi found in moldy maple bark, moldy malt, moldy wood chips and redwood dust, cheese mold, and paprika dust. There are various fungi, as well as amoeba, that can be found in ventilation systems. There are infectious and allergenic agents found in many workplaces, including health care settings and buildings with poor indoor air quality. Finally, there are chemicals such as phthalic anhydride and toluene diisocyanate, animal proteins found in bird droppings, and even bugs like the wheat weevil, that are linked to workplace respiratory diseases.

It's quite a list, isn't it? It might be helpful to split the list into two groups—inorganic gases, fumes, and chemicals in one; organic agents, excluding organic dusts discussed above, in the other—and take a look at them separately. Before we do that, however, it is important to understand how the particle size and composition of these various agents can affect the course of a respiratory disease and its effects on the human body.

The size and shape of airborne particles, as well as the concentration of the agent, length of exposure, and other factors determine where the particles will be deposited in the body. Particles first enter the human respiratory system through the nasopharyngeal area, the nose and mouth. Larger particles are trapped by the mucosa in the nasal passages. Smaller particles slip through initial entrapment and make their way into the tracheobronchial region, the trachea, bronchi, and bronchioles of the lungs. Even smaller particles penetrate farther to the pulmonary region, the areas in the lungs in which gas exchange occurs.

There are specific health effects associated with an agent's site of action in these different parts of the respiratory system. Typical health complaints when the nasopharyngeal region is affected include runny nose, sneezing, sore throat, unpleasant taste or smell, and tearing or stinging eyes. When the site of action moves from the upper airways in the head into the trachea and bronchi of the lungs, workers may experience coughing, increased amounts of sputum, and pain or tightness of the chest. Wheezing and shortness of breath may also be prominent. When the pulmonary region is affected, damage to the lungs resulting in fluid retention (edema) may occur. This causes extreme shortness of breath, cyanosis (a telltale condition in which the person's lips and nails take on a bluish discoloration due to the lack of oxygen in the blood), and collapse. Death can result from pulmonary edema.

The fate of these particles and how they affect the human body is also determined by their chemical composition and properties. These factors will influence how fast the particle is dissolved or absorbed in respiratory tract tissue, which will, in turn, affect how the body responds to these invaders.

Inorganic gases and fumes affect a large number of workers in various workplaces. Some of these common gases and fumes, and the occupations that may come in contact with them, are listed below.

- **Ammonia**—acetyline workers, aluminum workers, ammonia and ammonia salts workers, bronzers, chemical laboratory workers and chemical manufacturers, compressed gas workers, dry cleaners, electroplaters, farmers, fertilizer workers, glass cleaners, ice and ice cream makers, janitors, metal extractors, paper makers, perfume makers, photographic film makers, rayon makers, refrigeration workers, rubber workers, sewer workers, shellac makers, sugar refiners, tanners, and varnish makers

- **Chlorine**—aerosol propellant makers, bleachers, broom makers, carpet makers, chlorine workers, disinfectant makers, dye makers, flour bleachers, gasoline additive workers, gold extractors, ink makers, laundry workers, paper bleachers, photographic workers, plastic makers, sewage treaters, submarine workers, swimming pool maintenance workers, and water treaters
- **Hydrogen Sulfide**—animal fat and oil processors, artificial flavor makers, asphalt storage workers, blast furnace workers, brewery workers, cable splicers, cellophane makers, chemical laboratory workers and teachers, cistern and septic tank cleaners, dye makers, felt makers, fish-processing workers, fur dressers, glue makers, lithographers, livestock farmers, manhole and trench workers, metallurgists, miners, photoengravers, silk makers, soap makers, sulfur spa workers, textile printers, tunnel workers, and wool pullers
- **Mercury**—amalgam makers, barometer and thermometer makers, battery makers, boiler makers, calibration instrument makers, ceramics workers, chemical laboratory workers, dentists and dental technicians, drug makers, electroplaters, embalmers, explosive makers, fireworks makers, fur preservers and processors, histology technicians, insecticide makers, jewelers, lamp makers (fluorescent), neon light makers, photographers, silver extractors, taxidermists, and wood preservative makers
- **Sulfur Dioxide**—brewery workers, diesel engine operators and repairmen, firemen, food bleachers, foundry workers, fumigators, furnace operators, glass makers, meat preservers, oil processors, ore smelter workers, paper makers, petroleum refinery workers, preserva-

tive makers, sugar refiners, sulfuric acid makers, wicker ware bleachers, wine makers, and wood bleachers

Obviously, this list is not meant to encompass every occupation in which exposures to these agents is possible but is only a representative sample.

It is particularly difficult to track down organic agents that can cause respiratory diseases, because in most cases they are invisible to the naked eye. How would a secretary working in an office building possibly know that the heating and cooling system in the building is contaminated by bacteria that can cause respiratory illness? There are no odors and no outward signs that would warn her of her health risk.

Problems become more apparent in modern buildings that are constructed as sealed systems; that is, their windows serve to allow in light but not air. The air inside the building is recycled and filtered to varying degrees, with little, and sometimes no, outside air entering the system. How much fresh air enters the building is determined by the system's dampers, which could be set in any position from fully open to completely closed, although NIOSH recommends that they never be completely closed. The filtering process may be adequate for large particulates that could be in the air, but it is probably insufficient to filter out bacteria. Certain harmful bacteria can accumulate in the building's heating, ventilation, and air-conditioning (HVAC) system and contaminate it. As these bacteria are circulated through the system, people in the building are treated to breathing in a lungful or two.

This problem with indoor air quality, in which bacteria and other agents such as the proteins from pigeon droppings contaminate the air supply of a sealed building, has been dubbed "sick building syndrome," although the name is a misnomer since the building is not sick. The problem is with the air inside it.

The World Health Organization (WHO) estimates that as many as 30 percent of all commercial buildings show some signs of poor indoor air quality.[14]

Contaminants that affect indoor air quality may be produced within the building or drawn in from the outside and involve a host of agents. Mold and mildew, growing in the moisture in the air-conditioning system's drip pans, humidifiers, ductwork, and coils, can contribute to poor indoor air quality, as can dust and dirt in the system. Insecticides and fumigants that are not properly vented out of the building can be a problem. Sometimes solvents and cleaners used in the building by custodial services, or work materials used by the employees, can leave behind irritating fumes and residues. This may also be true for materials employees use on the job (think of the odors that teachers who still run mimeograph machines encounter). Outside agents like pollen, dust, fungal spores, industrial pollutants, and vehicle exhaust are other contributors to this syndrome. Odors from nearby Dumpsters, unsanitary debris near the outdoor air intake, and exhaust from the building that is drawn back into itself add to poor indoor air quality. Even the very soil upon which the building stands can pose an indoor air quality problem as radon, leakage from underground storage tanks, contaminants from previous site usage (a landfill, for example), or pesticides and lawn fertilizers find their way into the ventilation system. In one strange example, a nurse sued the hospital that employed her because she was breathing in helicopter exhaust fumes that entered the building through the intake vents located on the roof near the helicopter landing pad.[15]

One of the earliest documented cases of sick building syndrome resulted in a respiratory disease known as "Legionnaires' disease," because it struck delegates to a 1976 American Legion convention in Philadelphia. This incident focused awareness on unhealthful indoor air quality.

The symptoms experienced by persons working in buildings with indoor air quality problems are wide-ranging and include: headache; nausea; fatigue; shortness of breath; dizziness; eye, nose, and throat irritation; sinus congestion; and coughing and sneezing. These symptoms, however, are common to many other ailments unrelated to poor indoor air quality, so it is difficult to link their origins specifically to agents in the workplace. As an example, although most of us have experienced fatigue at work at one time or another, it is inaccurate to say that our fatigue was always caused by something in the air. Also, individuals have varying degrees of sensitivity to the causative agents. One individual may feel sick while most of his colleagues may not. Sometimes this reaction gives the false impression that the affected person may be faking his illness simply to get out of working. This misunderstanding could result in the actual problem never being discovered, or even investigated, since a supervisor could think the illness was the product of a lazy employee's vivid imagination. Worker dissatisfaction and conflict with management may result from this situation.

When workers complain about indoor air quality in a building, their complaints are frequently "something smells bad around here." But once again, we are all different creatures and even perceive odors differently, so the issue may still not be easily solved. The problem may also be intermittent so that a worker's complaint about an odor on Monday might seem imaginary to a supervisor who does not smell it on Tuesday.

Another common complaint is dust. Workers will assume that dust on windowsills, in storage areas, on computer screens, or on the tops of cabinets and desks poses a health hazard to them. Certainly, stirring up dust can produce coughing and sneezing, but this is more a mechanical reaction to an irritant than it is the onset of an actual respiratory disease. In fact, OSHA's dust standard is so liberal that at the level in which the agency states there may be a health risk, the dust would have to be so thick that the affected individual would have difficulty seeing more than a few feet in front of him! As you can probably guess, this standard was written for industries, such as construction and mining, where thick dust impairs visibility and poses a severe safety problem that could lead to fires and explosions. Still, even in an office setting the presence of dust will be perceived by some workers as an unhealthful situation, despite the fact that most homes are probably dustier than offices.

The problem of poor indoor air quality is not restricted to buildings, however. Any sealed area with recirculating air—airplanes, trains, submarines—can harbor the same illnesses. In airplanes, for example, viruses such as the common cold, influenza, measles, mumps, chicken pox, shingles, and infectious mononucleosis can all be spread from an infected passenger to others. In one case, a three-hour ground delay of a Boeing 737 with a nonoperating ventilation system resulted in 72 percent of the passengers contracting influenza from an infected passenger.[16]

What complicates finding a solution for indoor air quality problems is that OSHA doesn't have any standards established to regulate indoor air quality. Further, the agency does not have standards for most of the agents that cause respiratory illnesses associated with poor indoor air quality. Without such standards in place, there is no mechanism for ensuring that exposures to these agents are kept to a safe level since OSHA has not determined what those levels may be.

Does this lack of standards mean that supervisors and

company executives should be ignoring their workers' complaints about indoor air quality? Certainly not, for the sake of maintaining content and productive workers, but it does indicate how difficult it is to enforce corrective action in the workplace when no legal standards exist. Without the force of law, many companies are reluctant to enact safety and health measures that could be costly and that may adversely affect their profits.

It's important to pause here a moment to explain how exposure limits are determined and what they actually tell you in terms of health hazards. Both OSHA and NIOSH assign either a ceiling limit, a short-term exposure limit (STEL), a permissible exposure limit (PEL), or any combination of the three to nearly one thousand chemicals; only OSHA's standards carry the weight of law, however, and are enforced through legal action. NIOSH's limits are recommendations only, although OSHA frequently adopts them as standards.

Ceiling limits mean that at no time should the level of chemical exceed the amount determined as the maximum exposure level. The short-term exposure limit, generally set at 15 minutes, is the maximum allowable exposure to which an individual should be exposed over that time period. The permissible exposure limit is a long-term measurement, generally eight hours, and sets an *average* maximum exposure over that time period. As an example: If you were sitting in a hunting lodge for eight hours, using a defective space heater, and were exposed to carbon monoxide fumes that were measured at 50 ppm over that time period, you would have exceeded the OSHA permissible exposure limit of 35 ppm. If, however, you were exposed to carbon monoxide for two hours at 80 ppm and then went outside to hunt for six hours, your *average* exposure to carbon monoxide over eight hours is only 20 ppm, below OSHA's permissible limit of 35 ppm. The important thing to remember is that exposure limits have meaning only if we know how long the individual was exposed.

OSHA's exposure limits came under fire in 1989 when the agency adopted many of the American Conference of Governmental Industrial Hygienists' threshold limit values (TLVs). This action automatically assigned exposure limits to 164 new substances and reduced the limits on 212 others. Although OSHA's intentions were good, these new limits were challenged in court by industry associations and the AFL-CIO, who said that they were not supported by scientific evidence and that the permissible exposure limits were not protective enough. They also claimed that OSHA followed improper rule-making procedures in adopting the new PELs. The court ruled against OSHA. The agency was denied a new hearing, leaving its only legal recourse an appeal to the Supreme Court. The appeal was never filed and most PELs were rolled back to 1970 OSHA standards, where they remain today.

In the last few years, it was suggested that OSHA consider reviewing their standards on more than three hundred substances selectively, taking into consideration the number of workers exposed to a particular substance, the seriousness of the health effects, the data available for a quantitative risk assessment, and the agency's ability to conduct a feasibility analysis. The work is still ongoing and probably will be for a long time.

As common as respiratory illnesses caused by poor indoor air quality may be, there are other more debilitating respiratory diseases in the workplace, some of which just don't seem to go away.

Occupational asthma is a respiratory disease that can be found in many workplaces. Baker's asthma, which dates back to antiquity, is one of the most prevalent occupational asthmas, occurring in forms severe enough to cause fatalities. Flour dust is commonly implicated, but it is actually specific organic molecules within the dust that cause the disease. Two common allergens are wheat antigen and fungal alpha-amylase.

In 1996, six cases of physician-diagnosed occupational asthma in cosmetologists working with artificial fingernails caused the Colorado Department of Health to request assistance from NIOSH in evaluating and controlling nail salon technician exposures.[17] Methyl methacrylate, a substance also used in orthopedic surgery as bone cement, was previously used by cosmetologists to form artificial fingernails. The substance was found to cause dermatitis in both technicians and customers, central nervous system depression, eye irritation, and asthma and was banned for use in nail products by the U.S. Food and Drug Administration in 1974. Its chemical replacement, ethyl methacrylate, is toxicologically similar and may potentially be capable of inducing the same health afflictions, including asthma. It is possible that asthma may be occurring at levels below ethyl methacrylate's recommended limits, bad news for approximately 190,000 nail technicians using the substance.

Tuberculosis

Tuberculosis (TB) is one of the deadliest respiratory diseases in the world and has a long and tragic history. Formerly called consumption, tuberculosis is a common cause of death worldwide.

In nineteenth-century New England, in fact even into the early decades of the twentieth century, tuberculosis occurred with alarming frequency among silk and lace weavers. The disease was spread through the practice of wetting and sucking thread into weaving shuttles, a practice morbidly called the "kiss of death." In 1911, Massachusetts, Connecticut, and Rhode Island passed laws that prohibited the introduction of shuttles that required the use of lips or mouth in threading.

Tuberculosis is caused by the bacterium *Mycobacterium tuberculosis*, which is passed through the air when a person with an active case of tuberculosis coughs, sneezes, speaks, or sings. A cough that persists for three weeks or more could be an early sign of tuberculosis, especially if there are other symptoms such as fatigue, night sweats, and weight loss. People who are often in crowded, poorly ventilated places—an ideal environment for tuberculosis bacilli—are at a greater risk of contracting the disease than the general public. Individuals who have a compromised immune system as a result of AIDS or other diseases are the most vulnerable to tuberculosis infection.

OSHA estimates that as many as 13 million adults in the United States are currently infected with TB, and about 5.3 million workers in more than 100,000 hospitals, homeless shelters, long-term facilities for the elderly, detention facilities, laboratories, and other work settings are exposed to a high risk of tuberculosis.[18]

Since tuberculosis is a highly contagious disease, it can be communicated to individuals in any workplace, but the highest risk is still among physicians, nurses, and medical laboratory workers, all of whom have daily potential for contact with infected individuals. For example, 5 of 16 emergency workers in a Dallas hospital who were infected by a tuberculosis patient developed the disease; a sixth worker was infected by a coworker.[19] Over a 15-month period in an Atlanta hospital, 30–48 percent of the susceptible nursing staff and clerks on two wards were infected by a tuberculosis patient; eight developed active cases of the disease.

Other professions with an increased risk of exposure to the disease include miners, migrant farmworkers, zoo employees, prison guards, social workers, and those who work with the impoverished and derelict (as much as 7 percent of the homeless population have active cases of tuberculosis).

"While the rate of active TB in the general population has declined overall during the past 40 years, the risk for the workers who care for clients and patients infected with TB continues to be high, and in some areas is growing," said U.S. Labor Secretary Alexis Herman.

"Of even greater worry now," she said, "is the emergence of a new and deadly form of the disease that is resistant to current treatment. Infection with these multi-drug-resistant strains can lead to severe lung damage and is often fatal."[20]

While no health care worker would deliberately attempt to contract an occupational disease, there is sometimes a fatalistic attitude among these workers that the possibility of winding up with tuberculosis or some other disease as a result of their work is just one of those things—it comes with the territory. This is a dangerous attitude and foolhardy.

The rise in the number of AIDS cases in this country and worldwide is responsible, in part, for the rise of tuberculosis cases among health care workers. Since AIDS patients, by the very nature of their affliction, have little immunity to infectious diseases, they are particularly susceptible to tuberculosis. Health care workers and social workers who have AIDS patients as clients or patients are, therefore, at an increased risk of developing tuberculosis.

As the result of an upward turn in the number of tuberculosis cases reported nationwide, a coalition of labor unions petitioned OSHA in August 1993 for a permanent standard to control occupational exposures to the disease.[21] Although the Centers for Disease Control and Prevention (CDC) already had tuberculosis guidelines in place, there was no legal standard. OSHA could only enforce the guidelines under its "general duty clause," a catchall for enforcing corrective actions of dangerous safety and health conditions for which there is no standard. This is a strategy often used by OSHA but one that is easily challenged in court. Petitioning OSHA meant that if the agency agreed to develop a standard, the newly established standard would have the force of law behind it and could thus be enforced. Some of the unions included in the petition to OSHA were the American Federation of Government Employees; American Federation of State, County and Municipal Employees; American Federation of Teachers; Local 1199 National Health and Human Services Employees Union; and the Service Employees International Union.

It wasn't until 1998 that OSHA began public hearings on the agency's proposed standard. It is estimated that the proposed standard would prevent between 21,000 and 25,000 infections per year and save $89 million to $116 million in medical costs for the treatment of tuberculosis and lost production caused by employee absence from work and disabilities associated with active cases of the disease.

Some of the sections of the proposed standard call for exposure control, work practices and engineering controls, respiratory protection, medical surveillance, hazard communication and training, and proper record-keeping.

The exposure control section of the proposed standard requires employers to devise a plan to identify employees who have an occupational risk of contracting tuberculosis and to help them understand and minimize that risk. The plan must include exposure determination, a means of providing employees with information about individuals with suspected or confirmed infectious tuberculosis, information about ventilation, and procedures for reporting an exposure incident.

Other sections contain provisions for segregating individuals with suspected or confirmed tuberculosis in isolation rooms and for the use of respirators, not just surgical masks, by workers who are in contact with infected individuals. In addition, there are rules for medical evaluations, postexposure follow-up, and periodic tuberculin skin testing of workers with a potential exposure to the disease. Employers will be required to use proper signage to warn employees of exhaust systems that may harbor *Mycobacterium tuberculosis*, as well as laboratories where the bacteria may be present, and to label isolation rooms and other areas in which there are infected individuals.

A Breath of Fresh Air

As you can see, respiratory disease in the workplace is a common but very complicated issue. The variety of diseases, ranging in severity from simple sinus congestion to those causing death, brought on by an army of diverse agents makes it difficult for workers to understand the dangers in their workplaces and to protect themselves against them.

As always, knowledge is the best way to protect your health. You should understand which work practices pose a particular health risk and you should know how to perform those tasks safely. Material Safety Data Sheets (MSDS) must be available for your review when hazardous substances that require such data are used in the workplace. You have the right and the responsibility to read the data and learn about these substances. Representative Joseph Kennedy of Massachusetts introduced a bill on November 8, 1997, that would require the

Environmental Protection Agency (EPA) to publish a list of common indoor air pollutants and provide voluntary guidelines to help employers and building owners reduce occupational exposures.[22] This information could help you understand indoor air quality problems in your workplace.

The best way to reduce workplace exposures to respiratory diseases is to remove or minimize the effect of the offending agents. Improved general ventilation can help in removing many of the irritant agents associated with "sick building syndrome." The same type of controls employed in textile mills and other industries where fibers and dusts may accumulate can help reduce harmful exposures of these agents. Simple modifications of tools, such as a vacuum hose attached to an orbital sander in woodworking, remove dust right at the site and go a long way toward reducing worker exposures to dusts.

In addition to improved engineering controls, sometimes simply ensuring that the ventilation system is kept clean and dry can eliminate bacteria, molds, and fungi. In fact, this recommendation is part of OSHA's proposed indoor air quality standard. In construction and other industries where silica dust is a problem, it has been shown that exposures to the dust can be greatly reduced simply by wetting it down so that it is not airborne.

Obviously, not all disease-causing agents can be completely removed from the workplace by engineering controls and changes in work practices. Health care settings, especially in regard to tuberculosis patients, are examples of these types of workplaces. In their daily activities doctors, nurses, aides, and laboratory technicians may all come in contact with patients with active tuberculosis. It is important for those professionals to carefully follow protective measures guidelines, including the wearing of gowns, gloves, and respirators and surgical masks in order to protect themselves from infection. As scary as these precautions may seem to the patient and his family, they are necessary to protect others.

A quick word about respirators is needed here. A respirator is a device that fits securely over the nose and mouth and uses a filter to screen out certain substances from the inhaled air. In most cases, respirators are used as a last resort, only after engineering controls and changes in work practices have failed to correct the problem. OSHA estimates that anywhere from 2.6 to 7 million workers rely on respirators to protect them from respiratory disease. Respirators are effective when used properly and when the equipment is properly maintained. Any workplace in which respirators are required should have in place a respiratory protection program to ensure that workers know how to use and maintain their equipment. OSHA requires that a minimal acceptable program includes inspection for worn and damaged parts, regular cleaning and disinfection, and storage in a clean and sanitary location. The agency also requires a written program detailing standard operating procedures for the proper selection and use of respirators, which come in all sizes. Each worker should be fit-tested so that the respirator works for their particular facial structure.

For workers who smoke, occupational respiratory ailments can be much more serious. Smoking is strongly associated with many lung diseases, including chronic bronchitis, emphysema, and lung cancer. Moreover, smoking has an additive effect on the risk of chronic bronchitis in workers exposed to coal mine and other dusts, and it acts synergistically with asbestos to increase the risk of lung cancer. Evidence also indicates adverse health effects for those who are exposed to secondhand smoke. Many employers already prohibit smoking in the workplace, but if you're one of those who go outside to smoke and come back in to work, you're still rolling the dice on your health. So, if you haven't already, quit smoking; help make a safer workplace for you and your colleagues.

References

1. Moran, John B. 1997. "Silica Update: National Conference to Eliminate Silicosis." *Applied Occupational and Environmental Hygiene* 12:9.
2. Ibid.
3. Ibid.
4. Ibid.
5. U.S. Department of Health and Human Services. 1986. *Occupational Respiratory Diseases.* Washington, D.C.: U.S. Government Printing Office.
6. Ibid.
7. Ryan, G. et al. 1996. "A Longitudinal Study of an American Public Building Following Asbestos Removal." *Applied Occupational and Environmental Hygiene* 11:12.
8. Occupational Safety and Health Administration. 1998. Internet *News Release* July 18.
9. Occupational Safety and Health Administration. 1998. Internet *News Release* May 13.
10. Ibid.
11. Mokhiber, Russell. 1989. *Corporate Crime and Violence: Big Business Power and the Abuse of the Public Trust.* San Francisco: Sierra Club Books.
12. National Institute for Occupational Safety and Health. 1986. *Proposed National Strategies for the Prevention of Leading Work-Related Diseases and Injuries: Occupational Lung Diseases.* Cincinnati: NIOSH.
13. Korczynski, R.E. 1997. "Dust Exposure and Ventilation Control in the Crematorium." *Applied Occupational and Environmental Hygiene* 12:2.
14. American Industrial Hygiene Association. 1998. *The Synergist* 9:5.
15. Ibid.

16. Hocking, M.B. 1998. "Indoor Air Quality: Recommendations Relevant to Aircraft Passenger Cabins." *AIHA Journal* 59:7.
17. Spencer, Amy Beasley et al. 1997. "Control of Ethyl Methacrylate Exposures During the Application of Artificial Fingernails." *AIHA Journal* 58:3.
18. American Conference of Governmental Industrial Hygienists. 1997. *ACGIH Today!* 5:7.
19. Nicas, Mark. 1998. "A Risk/Cost Analysis of Alternative Screening Intervals for Occupational Tuberculosis Infection." *AIHA Journal* 59:2.
20. American Conference of Governmental Industrial Hygienists. 1997. *ACGIH Today!* 5:7.
21. American Industrial Hygiene Association. 1998. *The Synergist* 9:5.
22. American Industrial Hygiene Association. 1998. *The Synergist* 9:1.

CHAPTER 5

Dr. Jekyll and Mr. Hyde

Mike stood at the sink, vigorously scrubbing away the last dab of paint from his hands. He was tired; this last job had been a big one—a twelve room house on the east side—and the owner never seemed to know *exactly* what shade of blue she wanted. He felt that familiar headache coming on.

Someone knocked lightly on the bathroom door. "Daddy?"

He stopped washing his hands and lifted his head, his unsmiling face looking back at him from the mirror.

"Daddy, I have to go," a small voice said from beyond the door. Kelly, his 5-year-old.

He sighed. "Just a minute."

He rinsed his hands under the tap. He could feel a tightening in his skull, like someone stretching a steel band around it.

"Daddy?"

Mike grabbed the doorknob and flung the door open, his wet hands dripping on the floor. The door banged against the wall, startling the little girl standing in the hall.

"Damn it, Kelly, I told you in a minute, didn't I?"

The girl took a step back from him, afraid of the look in his eyes.

"Kelly, what's going on up there?" Maggie called from the kitchen downstairs.

As though his wife's voice were a hypnotist's wake-up command, Mike was suddenly aware of his frightened daughter standing there.

He bent down to her. "Kelly," he said, "I'm sorry. I didn't mean it. Here, come to Daddy." He held his arms wide for her.

Kelly hesitated, then let herself be hugged.

Mike held his daughter for a few moments, then released her. "Go ahead, you can use the bathroom now. I'll see you downstairs in a bit."

She closed the door.

He stood in the hall and let his body sag against the wall. He felt terrible about yelling at his daughter. He didn't know what had triggered his anger; it just happened. The pain in his head was lessening now, almost gone, but he knew it would only be a matter of time before it returned again.

He slowly made his way downstairs.

"What happened up there?" Maggie said. She looked at her husband and saw the pain in his eyes. "The headache again?"

He nodded.

"Mike, don't you think you should . . ."

"Please, Maggie, not now." He sank into one of the kitchen chairs.

"I only want to . . ."

He banged his fist on the table. A saltshaker did a little dance and rolled off the table.

"Maggie, not now!"

She didn't say anything further but simply turned to the stove where she had started dinner.

He sat at the table, his head propped up in one hand. He watched Maggie's back but couldn't bear to say anything to her. Just what the hell was wrong with him?

Mike would never have thought that his uncharacteristic behavior was brought on by the use of workplace solvents that were slowly poisoning his nervous system, but that was the case and he was not alone. In fact, disorders of the nervous system that result from toxic exposures encountered in the workplace have been known for almost two thousand years and have affected countless numbers of workers worldwide.

In the first century, Pliny discovered palsy among workers exposed to lead dust. In the 1800s, it was discovered that French workers who manufactured rubber products in small cottage industries exhibited bizarre psychoses that were traced to their exposures to carbon disulfide. When Lewis Carroll introduced his jittery, irritable, and apprehensive Mad Hatter in *Alice's Adventures in Wonderland*, he was bringing to life the phrase "mad as a hatter," and depicting the ubiquitous occupational neurological disorders (hatter's shakes) suffered by hat makers who used mercury in the process.

In the 1960s and early 1970s, Japanese workers exposed to the chemical acrylamide exhibited peripheral neuropathy, a disease of the nerves characterized by numbness and tingling in the feet or hands, followed by clumsiness or incoordination due to both sensory and motor changes. Since 1970, at least three significant outbreaks of neurotoxicity have occurred among workers as a result of exposure to chemicals: peripheral neuropathy from methyl-n-butyl ketone (MBK) and 2-t-butylazo-2-hydroxy-5-methyl hexane (BHMH) in manufacturing operations; and tremors, personality changes, and disturbances in vision and walking in workers using the pesticide chlordecone.[1]

The Problem

In 1983, OSHA listed neurotoxic disorders among the top ten leading causes of work-related disease and injury. There were several reasons for this: the sheer number of potentially toxic chemicals in the workplace, the number of workers exposed to these chemicals, the sensitivity of the human nervous system to such toxins, and the importance of an intact nervous system for daily functions.

It is estimated that 8 million workers may be exposed to neurotoxic agents full-time as a result of their job.[2] This is not to say that all 8 million experience neurotoxic effects, but the potential is certainly there when exposure levels become excessive. In addition, there are many more workers who are exposed to high levels of these agents on a short-term basis.

Neurotoxic agents affect both the peripheral nervous system (the nerves in the extremities), and the central nervous system (primarily the brain and spinal cord). The effects on the body are very different at each site.

Peripheral neuropathy, with its numbness, tingling, and incoordination, can leave a worker partly or fully impaired, depending upon the severity of the disease. The result, of course, is that the worker may no longer be able to perform his work tasks properly, if at all.

Other disorders of the peripheral nervous system caused by neurotoxicants include ataxia (irregular body movements); Parkinsonism, a condition that mimics the fine tremors of the head and extremities caused by Parkinson's disease; and a variety of nonspecific complaints such as motor weakness, weight loss, fatigue, and cramps.

The neurotoxic effects on the central nervous system occur with a broader range of chemicals, present more varied forms of disturbances, and are less readily recognized. Some of the most striking central nervous system disorders are those that are related to personality and cognitive functions. Memory impairment is seen in exposures to arsenic, carbon disulfide, lead, and manganese while carbon disulfide and manganese can also cause emotional instability and acute psychosis. Irritability, poor memory, and the inability to concentrate are some of the symptoms associated with neurasthenia, a disease caused by exposures to several chemicals, including acrylamide, arsenic, lead, MBK, mercury, and styrene. High concentrations of methylene chloride produce delusions and hallucinations, while psychoses and suicidal tendencies have resulted from exposures to manganese and carbon disulfide.

Unless thoroughly investigated, some of these disorders seem to have causes other than neurotoxicants, and may seem quite benign. Female workers at a telephone assembly plant in New Mexico complained of always being tired and irritable, of being depressed or anxious. They were considered by management to be malingering, as their symptoms were obviously "female problems." In fact, the workers had a history of several years' exposure to workplace solvents and were actually suffering from neurasthenia.[3]

Cognitive disorders as a result of workplace exposures to neurotoxic agents can result in shortened attention span, lack of alertness, or loss of memory. These effects have obvious safety implications and pose a hazard, not only for the affected individual, but for his coworkers as well.

Other central nervous system disorders that may potentially occur are:

Myoclonus—twitching or spasms of the muscles brought on by exposures to benzene hexachloride and mercury

Opsoclonus—jerky eye movements caused by chlordecone

Constricted visual fields or impaired visual acuity—a result of exposure to mercury, methanol, or n-hexane

Nystagmus—involuntary, cyclical movement of the eyeball caused by mercury exposures

Color vision loss—from styrene

Seizures—brought on by lead, organic mercurials, organotin compounds, or organochlorine insecticides

Tremors—caused by carbon disulfide, chlordecone, DDT, manganese, and mercury

Ataxic gait—irregular movements while walking, a result of exposure to acrylamide, chlordane, chlordecone, DDT, n-hexane, manganese, methylmercury, MBK, and methyl chloride

Impaired psychomotor function—from organophosphate insecticides, mercury, carbon disulfide, lead, styrene, perchloroethylene

Cranial neuropathy—from carbon disulfide and trichloroethylene

Bladder neuropathy—caused by exposure to dimethylaminopropionitrile (DMAPN)

Compounding the effects of workplace exposures to neurotoxins is the fact that many of these agents are also commonly found outside the job, at home perhaps, in hobbies and medication. Ethyl alcohol is one of the most common neurotoxicants and is frequently found in the home medicine cabinet as rubbing alcohol. A variety of neurotoxic solvents are found in glues, paints and stains, degreasers and nail polish remover, all of which are used widely outside the workplace. In addition, exposures to neurotoxic agents can occur from outdoor or community sources such as waste dumps, accidental toxic spills, and power-plant emissions. All these exposures can add to the neurotoxic effects a worker may experience from workplace exposures.

Still, the greatest potential for exposure to these agents is in the workplace and there are many horror stories to illustrate that point, especially when we are talking about organic solvents.

Organic solvents are a group of volatile compounds or mixtures that are relatively stable chemically and exist in the liquid state at temperatures of approximately 0° to 250°C (32° to 482°F). The volatility of organic solvents creates another serious problem in addition to their neurotoxicity; in 1989, a worker in an Ohio chemicals packaging company dropped a bottle of carbon disulfide that burst into flames when it was exposed to air. The worker was severely burned in the flash fire, two others were also injured, and five hundred people from businesses in a quarter-mile radius of the facility were evacuated.[4]

Organic solvents may enter the body through a number of pathways. They can be inhaled when they are volatized, as in spray painting, absorbed through the skin, or accidentally ingested as a result of unsanitary work practices (failing to wash hands before eating, nail biting, or putting hands to mouth when coughing or sneezing).

Typical organic solvents include a variety of hydrocarbons, ketones, esters, amines, alcohols, aldehydes, and ethers.

In more common terms, solvents are substances routinely used in paints, adhesives, glues, coatings, and degreasing and cleaning agents. They are also used in the production of dyes, polymers, glass, plastics, textiles, printing inks, agricultural products, and pharmaceuticals. Some typical organic solvents are carbon disulfide, n-hexane, methyl-n-butyl ketone, toluene, and trichloroethylene. In 1984, the United States International Trade Commission estimated that there were 49 million tons of industrial solvents produced that year.[5]

Organic solvents pose a potential health risk to any

worker using or manufacturing paints, varnishes, lacquers, stains, paint removers, glues, degreasers, cleaning agents, rubber cement, and rubber solvent. Shoemakers are exposed to the organic solvent trichloroethylene (in shoe adhesives), as are dry cleaners. Toluene is found in the production of benzene and gasoline and poses a problem for workers exposed to auto or airplane fuels.

An article in a 1989 issue of *Journal of Occupational Medicine* discussed the case of three workers who were sent to clean out a deactivated 30,000-gallon closed tank that had been previously used to store waste oils.[6] The company that owned the tank had decided to put it back into use and it had been vented to the open air at least two weeks before the workers—a welder and two assistants—climbed inside to clean it. The tank was not tested to see if it contained any residual gases or fumes since it had already been aired out. The welder worked less than ten minutes cleaning out some sludgy goop from the bottom of the tank before he became confused and asked for help. He was taken to the plant's first-aid station. The other two workers remained in the tank, but they too became confused and disoriented. All three men were then taken to a hospital emergency room, where one was hospitalized.

Three months later, the three workers were examined at the Occupational Medicine Clinic in Pittsburgh. Tests revealed that all the men exhibited damage to their vestibular systems (associated with balance). Each of the men demonstrated impairment in their ability to think, the degree of impairment varying among them. A year and a half after the initial incident, the workers were still impaired. Two of the men could not accurately process visual information quickly and would forget or distort the details of images they were shown. All three suffered from depression and insomnia.

Researchers determined that the workers' neurological disorders were a result of exposure to hydrocarbons in the tank. What was particularly alarming in this case was that such a short-term exposure produced such long-term effects.

The long-term neurological effects of organic solvents has also been demonstrated in workers exposed to trichloroethylene, a solvent commonly used in degreasers, paints, varnishes, lacquers, and in the dry cleaning industry. In a 1955 study by Swiss researcher E. Grandjean, levels of the solvent as low as 40 to 80 ppm in the air were responsible for loss of memory, emotional instability, and disorientation among exposed workers.[7] Grandjean recommended that workplace exposures to the solvent be kept below 40 ppm; even now, the OSHA standard for trichloroethylene is 100 ppm.

Perchloroethylene, similar to trichloroethylene, is the most commonly used (40,000 locations) dry-cleaning solvent in the United States. In addition to less serious health effects such as dizziness, headaches, and dermatitis, the chemical may be linked to esophageal, pancreatic, and urinary tract cancers. In 1995, the International Agency for Research on Cancer (IARC) classified perchloroethylene as a probable human carcinogen.

There is some disagreement among U.S. regulatory agencies when it comes to determining exposure limits to dangerous chemicals. There are three agencies and professional associations involved, and each of them uses different criteria to make their evaluations. A brief explanation here may be helpful in understanding these differences.

The Occupational Safety and Health Administration (OSHA), the National Institute for Occupational Safety and Health (NIOSH), and the American Conference of Governmental Industrial Hygienists (ACGIH) are the three U.S. organizations that determine and promulgate exposure limits for a wide range of chemicals and physical and biological agents found in the workplace. Though they all have the same end product, their philosophies and methods are quite different and need to be understood.

NIOSH is a government agency charged with researching and recommending solutions to occupational hazards. The agency's emphasis is placed entirely on worker safety and health; that is, it works to determine the safest standards and work practices for all workers at all times, usually without taking into consideration the economic costs that may result to an employer who implements the agency's *recommendations*. It is important to stress the word "recommendations." NIOSH does not have any legal authority to enforce occupational health laws and so can only recommend what it considers safe standards and practices in the workplace. NIOSH strives to create the ideal safe workplace through its recommendations, knowing full well that the actual workplace situation will probably fall short of its ideals.

OSHA is the government agency charged with determining safety and health standards that will serve as the law of the land. Although the agency frequently accepts NIOSH's research and recommendations and may adopt them as legal standards, the agency is under no obligation to do so. The agency does not perform research on health and safety problems, but it will investigate complaints in which it appears that safety and health standards have been violated. OSHA has the power to fine companies that do not adhere to its standards. In some circumstances criminal charges against the company and even individuals within that company may be brought by state or federal prosecutors.

OSHA works with both workers and companies to try to establish a balance between ideal safety-and-health standards and the economic reality of the workplace. It examines the cost of implementing safety standards and how that will affect a particular industry. Although OSHA is interested in maintaining the safety and health of the American workforce, it is also concerned about maintaining a healthy business economy, and so walks a fine line between the two, frequently drawing the ire of labor unions and activists who believe the agency favors the corporations. By comparison, NIOSH is sometimes seen as favoring the unions and individual workers, rather than the corporations.

ACGIH is a professional association of industrial hygienists that is over 50 years old and predates OSHA and NIOSH, both of which were established in 1970. The association's purpose is to recommend threshold limit values (TLVs) and biological exposure indices (BEIs) for workplace hazards that may affect *most* workers, as compared to NIOSH's *all* workers. Each year the association reviews its guidelines and revises them or develops new ones, then publishes the information in a handbook. This annual review allows ACGIH to be more quickly responsive to new research or changes in the workplace, much faster than OSHA, which can often be mired down for years trying to develop a single standard. As an example, OSHA first published an advance notice of a proposed standard for methylene chloride, a solvent used widely in the furniture-stripping industry, in 1986. It wasn't until 1997 that the final standard was established (in fairness to OSHA, at least part of the delay was political as the regulation was held up by a last-minute appropriations rider).

Even though OSHA initially adopted most of ACGIH's already existing recommendations as its first round of legal standards when the agency was formed, ACGIH itself does not have any legal authority to enforce standards.

Generally, ACGIH's recommendations fall somewhere

between those of NIOSH and OSHA. The association may be a bit more lenient than NIOSH and may concede that there are times when it is impractical to adhere to the ultimate standards.

In addition to United States agencies, most of the industrialized nations of the world have agencies that determine workplace standards, as does the United Nations' World Health Organization. Even though none of these agencies has any bearing on standards set in this country, it can be interesting to compare foreign standards with our own.

So, with three different U.S. agencies, each promoting their own set of standards, which often differ, how does a company know which one to use?

The answer is that it depends on what the company is trying to accomplish. If the company's goal is only to make sure that it is in compliance with the letter of the law relative to occupational safety and health, then merely complying with OSHA's standards would be enough.

Remember, however, that OSHA's standards are generally something of a compromise between workers and industry. There will be workers who will suffer workplace accidents or exposures to dangerous substances even at the OSHA-prescribed levels. Companies that understand this may strive for conformity to ACGIH guidelines, although they are not legally obligated to do that. The company may take this action in response to union demands for a safer workplace, to reduce its worker compensation payments, or simply as a matter of conscience.

It is doubtful that more than a few companies would try to conduct their business in accordance with NIOSH's recommendations. A company that did so would demonstrate the highest regard for the safety and health of every one of its workers and would incur any cost to ensure that safety. Pessimistic as it may sound, one would have to search long and hard to find a company with such impeccable moral standards.

The reality of the American workplace is that the majority of companies recognize OSHA standards as the law and do just enough to keep themselves compliant to the law, although they often break it and try to influence newly proposed standards or challenge them in court. The recent flap over OSHA's new standard for methylene chloride serves as an example.

Methylene chloride, one of the most common organic solvents, is widely used by about 237,500 workers at 92,000 work sites. Among other applications, it is used as a paint stripper and metal cleaner. Workers' exposures typically occur during degreasing and paint-stripping operations, while using ink solvents, and during construction remodeling or renovation.

In 1997, OSHA reduced its permissible exposure limit for methylene chloride from 500 ppm to 25 ppm and was soon challenged by two industry groups, the Halogenated Solvents Industry Alliance and the United Auto Workers. The industry alliance said the more stringent standard would be detrimental to the nation's small businesses because the implementation of the standard would be too expensive. The labor union, on the other hand, argued that workers would be afraid to report their symptoms to the company medical officer because they would then not be allowed to work and would lose their pay. The union said the OSHA standard was unacceptable because the medical restriction clause did not include a provision that would allow workers to report their illness without fear of losing their jobs.[8]

More to Think About

In an industrial area of Quebec, it was discovered that the incidence of Parkinsonism among the residents was two to five times higher than the rest of Quebec.[9] A study, led by researchers from the University of Quebec, examined 115 workers with an average employment history of 14 years employed in a large ferromanganese and silicomanganese alloy facility. These workers were exposed to manganese dust caused by manganese fumes and the crushing and screening of the metal. The study was a matched pair study, which means that the workers were compared one-on-one to other subjects recruited from the area with similar characteristics (age, height, weight, educational level, smoking status, and number of children).

After both groups were put through a battery of tests, it was shown that the manganese plant workers performed significantly more poorly than their counterparts on motor tasks involving rapidly alternating, coordinated movements of one or both hands. Even when surveyed off the job, the workers experienced more fatigue, adverse emotional states, memory loss, and nightmares than the nonworkers.

The symptoms that emerged among the workers in the study were remarkably similar to those described in classical manganism, a neurological disorder caused by exposures to manganese, which was first studied in 1837. Even more important, the study demonstrated that long-term exposure to manganese alters specific functions of the nervous system.

Other sources of manganese exposures are fertilizers, mining, welding, steel finishing, matches and fireworks, and dry cell batteries. In addition to manganese, other metals such as arsenic, lead, mercury, nickel, tellurium, thallium, and tin are also neurotoxicants depending on the level of exposure. The sources of workplace exposure for these metals are many and varied.

Arsenic—pesticides, smelters, seafood, well water, semiconductors, electroplating, and pigments

Lead—solder, lead shot, lead pipes, lead stained glass, leaded paint, pottery, smelters and foundries, insecticides, storage batteries, radiator repair and auto body shops, manufacture of cans

Mercury—farming, dental amalgams, pigments, photography, taxidermy, scientific instruments, electrical equipment, electroplating, felt making, and textiles

Nickel—paints, inks, alloys, coinage, electroplating, surgical instruments, nicad batteries, and mining

Tellurium—foundries, electronics, glazes and glass, semiconductors, rubber vulcanizers, and thermoelectric devices

Thallium—rodenticides, fungicides, special lenses, photoelectric cells, optical devices, and mercury and silver alloys

Tin—solder, silverware, fungicides, mining, canning, electronics, polyvinyl plastics, and coated wire

One of the most common and possibly most dangerous neurotoxicants on the list is lead, a metal that is ubiquitous in the environment, found in air, water, food, soil, dust, and gasoline. Since lead used to be an ingredient in most paints, workplace exposures to the metal are often incurred during sanding, stripping, cutting, and welding surfaces coated with lead-based paint, as in custodial work or renovation and demolition of old structures. In addition, artists working in stained glass, pottery, or painting with lead-based paints may also be exposed.

Once lead is inhaled or accidentally ingested, it accumulates in bone and soft tissues, with only a small amount being excreted in the urine. Consequently, lead levels build up in the body over time, resulting in lead poisoning. Since lead is stored in the bones for decades and slowly released into the body, adverse health effects may be seen long after exposure.

Lead poisoning has been found in the children of

workers exposed to lead. These workers may bring lead dust home on their bodies, clothing, tools, or other objects in the workplace, thus exposing their children. The risk to children is great since they often put their hands in their mouths and because their bodies absorb lead quickly. Some of the adverse health effects connected to lead exposures in children include behavioral changes such as increased distractibility and aggressiveness, significant decreases in intelligence quotient (IQ), increased academic failure, and brain damage. A NIOSH study examined thirty-one children of lead-exposed workers and compared them to a control group of nineteen children of nonexposed workers. The study showed that the children of exposed workers were six times more likely to have blood lead levels over the recommended limit than children of nonexposed workers.[10]

"Parents wouldn't take their children to a dangerous workplace. It's equally important that they do not bring the hazards of the workplace home to their families," said NIOSH Director Linda Rosenstock.[11]

While lead has adverse effects in the kidneys, the blood-forming system, and digestive and reproductive systems, we will concern ourselves here with its effects upon the nervous system.

Common symptoms of overexposure to lead include fatigue, sleep disturbances, headache, irritability, anxiety, aches and pains in bones and muscles, and decreased appetite. However, these symptoms are nonspecific and occur with a host of other minor ailments, so linking them to lead poisoning is not easy. Later findings may include decreased handgrip strength, fine tremors, and "wrist drop," a condition in which the hand drops downward at the wrist caused by damage to the radial nerve. Extreme overexposures to lead could result in seizure, coma, and even death, although because of more efficient material handling methods in the workplace and biological monitoring, life-threatening cases of lead poisoning are rare today. Still, lead exposures are common in industry and they should not be treated lightly; even in mild cases of lead poisoning the effects may not be reversible, even after lead levels in the bloodstream drop.

There has been some progress made in the last few decades in reducing lead exposures. Blood levels of lead in the general U.S. adult population (ages 20 to 74) dropped significantly between 1976 and 1991, from 13.1 µ/dl (micrograms of lead per deciliter of blood) to 3.0 µg/dl. This drop is largely credited to the reduction of lead in gasoline. Today, more than 98 percent of the adult population has blood lead levels less than 15 µg/dl. In the workplace, the U.S. Public Health Service has set a goal to eliminate by the year 2000 all occupational exposures to lead that result in blood lead levels greater than 25 µg/dl.

Some gases are also neurotoxicants. Carbon monoxide may be the best known, with exposures produced by poorly ventilated stoves and furnaces, acetylene welding, internal combustion engine exhaust, and enclosed areas such as mines and tunnels.

There are several neurotoxic gases commonly found in the health care industry. Ethylene oxide is routinely used to sterilize medical equipment and supplies while nitrous oxide, halothane, enflurane, isoflurane, and desflurane are used either as dental or surgical anesthetics. NIOSH has concluded that exposure to nitrous oxide causes decreases in mental performance, audiovisual ability, and manual dexterity. One must wonder how safe a surgical patient may be under these circumstances; the one word you do not want to hear from your surgeon is "whoops."

Knowledge Is Everything

As you can see, neurotoxicants occur in a myriad of forms across a broad spectrum of industries. There are so many—how can you protect yourself from their effects?

As always, the best defense is to be aware of the dangers of your workplace, especially in regard to the substances you encounter there. "Right-to-know" laws provide you with the necessary information to protect yourself and others.

As you should be aware of your workplace, you should also be aware of your individual situation within it. With neurotoxicants particularly, be aware of changes in your mental state. Do you feel "stressed out"? Having a "bad day"? Suffering headaches, irritability, loss of attention, "fuzzy" thinking? While everyone periodically experiences these things, a constant pattern of these traits may indicate that something else is going on in your workplace. Your symptoms may have an occupational source.

Also, keep in mind that neurotoxic effects can last a long time, even as a result of a relatively brief exposure, and that minor, annoying symptoms can be indicative of a more serious health problem. It is important to remember that chemical interactions may occur between substances to which you may be exposed in the workplace and chemicals you encounter in other aspects of your life. As examples, drug usage (both prescription and illegal), alcohol, and smoking all involve chemicals that may react in unexpected ways with workplace chemicals already in your body. Chemicals you use at home in hobbies, lawn care, cleaning, and other household tasks may do the same.

When workplace neurotoxic effects can be linked to certain substances, there are standard measures that a company should take to reduce its workers' exposures to them.

One method of reducing exposures is to substitute

benign substances for hazardous ones wherever possible. As an example, the substitution of water-based paints for solvent-based types would eliminate some exposures to dangerous solvents. Replacing equipment that may cause toxic exposures with machinery that will reduce or eliminate those exposures is another method. This was done in the process of spray-painting, where newly designed equipment reduced the dispersion of paint particles into the air.

Sometimes, an entire process can be substituted for a new one that reduces or eliminates toxic exposures. As an example, taping something that was formerly glued could reduce exposures to solvents in the glue. Isolating hazardous substances is another effective method of reducing toxic exposures. Paint spray booths are good examples of this method.

One of the easiest methods of reducing exposures is to ensure adequate ventilation in the workplace. The source of exposure should be enclosed as much as possible in order to shield other workers from being exposed to the chemical and to keep it from entering the air in the rest of the facility. Local exhaust ventilation, which removes gases and fumes at the immediate source, can greatly reduce these toxic exposures. The ventilation system should be as close as possible to the source of exposure, and it must have a velocity strong enough to adequately draw the toxic gases or particles into the system. The air flow should also be directed in such a manner as to draw gases or particles away from the exposed workers without drawing them past anyone else. Finally, routine maintenance of the ventilation system can go a long way toward keeping it running in top form and helping to keep exposures to a minimum.

It is important for a company to use its workers as consultants to the ventilation contractors who will install the system. Too often, systems are built without the input of the workers actually handling the toxic substances and the resulting ventilation system fails to adequately protect them or allow them to properly do their job. When that happens, the ventilation system will be circumvented by the very people it was supposed to help so that the job can get done.

Some job tasks may require you to wear respirators or masks in order to minimize your exposure to workplace neurotoxicants. For a discussion of respirators and masks, see Chapter Four.

Because of their scope and cost, the methods listed above require implementation by the company, rather than the workers, but you can still be involved in change. As a worker, you often know your workplace conditions better than management and your advice and suggestions can possibly result in a safer and more healthful workplace. There are different ways to make your voice heard—suggestion boxes, reports to supervisors, through union representatives—but no matter how you do it, it is important for you to know your workplace and speak up to improve it. Ultimately, you have to protect yourself.

References

1. National Institute for Occupational Safety and Health. 1988. *Proposed National Strategies for the Prevention of Leading Work-Related Diseases and Injuries*. Cincinnati: NIOSH.
2. Ibid.
3. Lappe, Marc. 1991. *Chemical Deception: The Toxic Threat to Health and the Environment*. San Francisco: Sierra Club Books.
4. *The Cincinnati Enquirer*. 1998. News article July 16.
5. National Institute for Occupational Safety and Health. 1987. *Organic Solvent Neurotoxicity*. Cincinnati: NIOSH.

6. Lappe, Marc. 1991. *Chemical Deception: The Toxic Threat to Health and the Environment.* San Francisco: Sierra Club Books.
7. Ibid.
8. American Conference of Governmental Industrial Hygienists. 1997. *ACGIH Today!* 5:2.
9. Mergler, D. et al. 1992. "Micromanganism: Early Nervous System Dysfunction Among Manganese Exposed Workers." *Proceedings of the 9th. International Symposium on Epidemiology in Occupational Health.* Cincinnati: NIOSH.
10. American Conference of Governmental Industrial Hygienists. 1997. *ACGIH Today!* 5:6.
11. Ibid.

CHAPTER 6

Is It All in Your Head?

Mark turned his company car into the driveway of the hotel, grateful for the rest the hotel would provide. Another tough day on the road, calling on the same old accounts again, begging for an order, even the hint of an order, anything he could exaggerate as "positive" in his report to his demanding boss. Maybe he was getting too old for the job, or maybe the competition was stronger, or maybe the economy was in a slump, he didn't know, but whatever the reasons, Mark felt his livelihood slipping away from him and he was scared.

As soon as he checked in, even before he went up to his room, he headed for the hotel lounge. A double scotch helped take the edge off and he began to feel a little more relaxed. Still, he couldn't help remembering his sales manager's dire predictions for the sales force. Several territories had already been consolidated and Mark was one of those who had acquired some additional territories. He didn't want more territory; he was having trouble making the quota in his own area as it was.

As if that wasn't enough pressure, his expanded territory meant that he was away from home a lot more, away from his wife and kids. He didn't like being away so much and he knew Michele was finding it difficult to take care of the children and the house all by herself. It seemed there was always something happening when he was not home. A leaking roof, a flat tire, measles, his son Lee picking a fight again, always something.

A second scotch helped him feel better.

After sitting in the lounge for an hour, he went upstairs to his room. He watched TV for a while, finding nothing of interest, then called home.

His wife's voice, faintly carried to him over two hundred miles, was weary. He feared the worst.

"Is something wrong?" he asked.

"No, I'm just tired. I had to chauffeur two of the kids to different soccer games, then take Diane to the library. I was going to go grocery shopping, but I ran out of steam. I just started running the bathwater when you called."

She did sound tired, and he felt guilty that he was not there to help.

"You'll be home tomorrow, right?" Michele said.

"Tomorrow? No. Harris canceled our appointment today and rescheduled. I'll be home a day late."

"Oh, no, Mark . . ."

It was then that he remembered Diane's piano recital was tomorrow night. He would not be there for her again.

"Mark, you promised."

He felt trapped. He could not get home to his daughter's recital, much as he would have liked to. He couldn't jeopardize his job. He felt a dull pain in his chest that hurt every time he breathed.

When Michele hung up a few moments later, Mark went back down to the bar. Maybe one more would help him forget.

The stress and anxiety that Mark experiences as a result of his job, along with his growing dependency on alcohol, are psychological disorders that can cripple his job performance and adversely affect his physical and mental health.

Because psychological disorders are so varied in nature and their causes complex, it is difficult to draw a clear picture of the occupational factors relevant to these disorders. Still, workplace experiences can have a pervasive influence, both good and bad, on our overall psychological and physical well-being and need to be examined. Several countries, recognizing the importance of good mental health in the workplace, have set up agencies to deal specifically with that health problem. In Japan, the Japan Productivity Center has a large division dedicated to workplace mental health, while the International Committee of Occupational Mental Health has over 350 members, mostly from the United Kingdom, Netherlands, Belgium, and the Scandinavian countries.

In Western society, so much of our lives are played out in the workplace that it becomes difficult for us to separate our private lives from our jobs. As a result, problems with our children and spouses that affect us mentally, as well as our own individual psychological foibles, are brought into the workplace. Conditions on the job may add even more to our psychological burdens.

Yet, the Protestant work ethic, for which American workers are famous, demands that we give a solid day's work to our employers, come hell or high water, sickness or health. This same ethic places a high premium on the value of work and the importance of, to paraphrase U.S. Army television ads, being all you can be.

We are identified by our jobs. When introduced to someone, the first question asked is "What do you do?" In this country, we know the other person is asking what your job is. Your answer will set up some preconceived notions about you in the other person's mind, some favorable, some not. The workplace and our jobs have a major psychological effect on who we are; workplace factors that can throw our psychological balance out of kilter can have a ripple effect throughout the other areas of our lives. Albert Camus, in *The Myth of Sisyphus*, summed it up succinctly when he wrote, "Without work, all life goes rotten, but when work is soulless, life stifles and dies."[1]

The Problem

What are we talking about when we say occupational psychological disorders? The expression "psychological disorders" connotes a category of problems encompassing a wide variety of social, behavioral, and biomedical conditions with diverse, and frequently unknown, origins. When we attach the "occupational" qualifier to the term, we are referring only to those conditions that develop in or can be affected by the workplace. As an example, schizophrenia and mental retardation are psychological states that develop independently of the workplace and are not usually affected by it, and so would not be considered occupational.

To keep things simple, most psychological disorders in the workplace fall under the general term "stress." The term is ambiguous, yet we all seem to recognize stress when we experience it, and understand how it feels.

Loosely defined, stress is a process through which an individual responds to stressors—stimuli, events, or conditions that affect the individual in some adverse way. These stressors may come directly from the physical environment surrounding the person or they may arise in the person's thoughts and feelings generated by his psychic and social environment. The individual's response to the stressors may be manifested physically, chemically, physiologically, psychologically, emotionally, or even metaphysically.

Each of us is confronted daily with innumerable stressors. How we react to them is highly idiosyncratic, determined by many factors, including genetics, past experiences, degree of sensitivity or vulnerability at that time, and the context in which the stressor is perceived. Each of us has a certain tolerance for accumulated stressors. Once that point is exceeded, we experience one or more of the manifestations typical of stress.

Stressors occur at home, in our private lives, in our family relationships, in our community, and at work. Some workers who are already subjected to stressors from other aspects of their lives may be at risk of becoming stressed when they come to work and encounter the unique stressors of their workplace. These stressed workers may themselves become stressors to their coworkers.

Workplace stressors are of many varieties. They may be found in disagreeable coworkers and supervisors, shift changes, deadlines and quotas, physical demands of the job, personal comfort on the job, personal safety, and many other conditions. One unusual workplace stressor was discovered in Germany among train drivers. It is estimated that each year one thousand people in Germany commit suicide by jumping or standing in front of trains.[2] According to Deutsche Bahn, the German national railway system, most train drivers can expect at least one suicide in their careers on the rails. The problem is so common that the railway system always has a driver on duty who has experience with train suicide. Additionally, a replacement driver will take the train the rest of the way after a suicide. In most cases, the driver will take a few days off after the incident, and if symptoms of stress occur can consult with one of twelve Deutsche Bahn psychologists.

The effects of stress on the human body range in severity and are predicated upon individual responses to stressors. Usually, the nervous system initiates physiologic changes in the body typical of the "fight or flight" response. Hormonal secretions will be affected. Prolonged stress may cause impairment of the immune system, resulting in heart disease, stroke, arthritis, and cancer.[3]

Stress can adversely affect the body directly, as in heart disease, or it can work indirectly by causing workplace accidents. An example of this is the 60-year-old paper cutter with a long history on the job, who suddenly developed hypertension.[4] His condition worsened, and after fainting while getting out of bed one morning, he was urged by the plant physicians to take an early retirement since his condition made it difficult for him to work safely at his job. After much hesitation and anxiety, the paper cutter decided to accept the favorable pension offered by the company. While the pension package was being put together, he continued to work, his misgivings increasing as he realized how empty his life would be without his job. With only three hours left in the last day on his job, despite all safety precautions, he cut off his right hand, his first injury on the job in thirty-two years.

The example of the paper cutter points out how stress can affect a worker in ways that cannot be predicted. Could the accident have been avoided? As long as the man was allowed to stay on the job, there was the possibility of an accident, despite his being intimately knowledgeable about the workings of his machinery and what it would take to override safeguards. The accident might have been avoided if the physicians who initially recognized the danger the man's condition presented to his safety on the job had transferred him to a desk job for his last few weeks. Sometimes, even in cases in which the psychological disturbance is identified, the situation can be made worse when company managers or health professionals fail to take the appropriate action.

Workplace accidents as a result of stress are also seen among workers who routinely change shifts. The frequent changes in work periods and sleep periods interfere with the worker's circadian rhythm, resulting in stress, fatigue, and a reduction in mental alertness. Night shift workers often have difficulty sleeping soundly during the day. They may experience micro-sleep, a condition in which they fall asleep for only a few seconds. This condition could be very dangerous if they micro-sleep while driving a car, or when using machinery. In addition to accidents, the stress of shift work has been linked to digestive disorders and increased evidence of heart attacks.

There are some psychological conditions caused by the workplace, however, that are more specific than stress and can develop into clinical disorders. These conditions include:

- **Affective disorders** such as anxiety, depression, and job dissatisfaction
- **Maladaptive behavioral and lifestyle patterns**
- **Chemical dependencies and alcohol abuse.**

While the number of those affected may be in question, the American Psychological Association does not dispute the role of occupational factors in psychological disorders and lists "occupational stress" in its *Diagnostic and Statistical Manual* as a major "psychological stressor."

In the 1970s, two Swedish studies showed that about one-fourth to one-third of workers in that country considered their work "stressful," or reported mild to high levels of stress while at work.[5] A 1984 study by the Canadian Mental Health Association showed that 60 percent of the workers in the study experienced "negative stress" at work in the previous year, and 35 percent reported "adverse psychological effects."[6]

It is a little easier to get an idea of the magnitude of psychological disorders in the workplace when we examine workers' compensation data. Generally, claims for psychological disorders that result from job experiences have been increasing. The State of California alone received 3,000-4,000 psychiatric injury claims in 1979, half of which received monetary awards.[7] A 1983 study by the California Workers' Compensation Institute showed that while claims for all other disabling injuries decreased by 10 percent from 1980 to 1982, claims for gradual mental stress doubled in that same time period ("gradual mental stress" is a term used by insurance companies that refers to cumulative emotional problems caused by adverse psychological conditions at work; it does not refer to emotional problems brought on by specific workplace incidents, such as witnessing an accident). The National Council on Compensation Insurance reported that the cost of workers' compensation for gradual mental stress in 1981–1982 surpassed the average cost of claims for other occupational diseases.

It is estimated that costs for psychological disorders, in terms of medical services, employment, and productivity, run in the tens of billions of dollars annually. Adding in the cost of physical health problems related to psychological disorders, such as hypertension, brings the bill up to $50-$100 billion annually.[8]

There are several factors in the workplace that can result in psychological disorders.

The workload and the work pace of a particular job can cause psychological disturbances. Surprisingly, it is not so much the amount of work or how fast that work must be done that affects workers as much as it is how much control workers believe they have over these functions. Evidence seems to indicate that control is the decisive factor in determining the health consequences of work demands. Adverse effects occur when workers do not feel their control is commensurate with the demands of the job. Think of Lucy Ricardo working at the candy conveyor belt in *I Love Lucy* and you get the idea.

Similarly, how much participation a worker has in the decision-making process relative to his job will affect his psychological well-being. Some studies have shown that mood disturbances, lowered self-esteem, and impaired supervisory relationships may result when workers feel left out of the decision-making process.[9]

Workload and work pace factors should not be treated lightly. Workers who cannot tolerate these factors may either crumble under the pressure or lash out. This may be what happened in the several reported cases of U.S. Postal Service workers committing murder in the workplace—"going postal," as the phenomenon has been termed.

The work schedule is also a factor in psychological disorders. Workers on rotating shifts or permanent night work are particularly susceptible to these disorders. It is theorized that the disruption of their circadian rhythms as well as the interference with normal social interaction caused by their odd hours could be at the heart of the problem.

Uncertainty about security or career issues can also pose health risks. Workers who do not know if they will have a job from one day to the next due to economic conditions, strikes, downsizings, plant closings, mergers, relocations, or job obsolescence may suffer from low job and life satisfaction, low self-esteem, and generally poor health. The same could be said for workers who feel they have been overlooked for promotion or are facing early retirement.

Uncertainty about one's role or job function, or conflict about those things, may result in psychological disorders. A worker who is asked to perform tasks he doesn't think are part of his job can experience lowered self-confidence, lower job satisfaction, and higher job tension. This would also apply to workers who do not fully understand their role and find out, usually a stressful minute too late, that they were responsible for something that didn't get done, or didn't get done properly. These factors have been linked to depressed mood, tension, anxiety, resentment, and increased heart rate and blood pressure.

Poor relationships with workplace colleagues, supervisors, and subordinates are another risk factor for psychological disorders, especially depression and job dissatisfaction. However, a 1982 National Institute for Occupational Safety and Health (NIOSH) study of one thousand male workers showed that these adverse health effects could be minimized when workers had the support of coworkers and supervisors.[10] Similarly, workers who have a supportive environment at home are better equipped to deal with workplace relationships in a healthy way.

The nature of the work task has considerable effect on psychological well-being. Tasks that are short-term and boring, with little mental stimulation or potential for creativity, and that require few skills, have been linked to job dissatisfaction and poor mental health.

While these factors may affect any one of us in the workplace, how we respond will differ markedly, depending upon personal parameters such as overall mental and physical health, and life events such as family problems, financial difficulties, and major life changes. Type A personality behavior, characterized by competitiveness, time urgency, and overcommitment, may be exacerbated in a stressful job, although there is the possibility that individuals with this type of personality deliberately seek out demanding jobs.

An interesting response to stress is a condition known

as *multiple chemical sensitivities*. This syndrome is characterized by the worker's sensitivity to many chemically unrelated substances at doses far below those determined to have a harmful effect on the general population. The multiple chemical sensitivities syndrome is just one of many medical problems that are collectively called "twentieth century disease," a term that includes many health problems associated with the impact of modern technology on the environment. The symptoms are varied, affecting several organ systems, and are recurrent. They cannot be traced to any single physiologic function.

Workers with multiple chemical sensitivities acquire their condition after they experience a documentable workplace exposure, illness, or injury that results in a noticeable, but usually acute, reaction. Then, for reasons still not understood, these workers will subsequently experience adverse effects of some kind to a wide variety of stimuli, many of which have no connection to their initial experience.

A typical example of multiple chemical sensitivities is the worker in his mid-fifties who worked in a chemical refinery plant and was involved in a series of chemical spills.[11] His exposure to toxic chemicals resulted in brief periods of medical leave after which he returned to work. After the fourth accident, however, the man complained of lingering symptoms and a lowered sensitivity to workplace chemicals; he would be bothered simply as he drove past the plant. In addition, he began to experience symptoms of sensitivity to environmental stimuli such as house paint or traffic fumes. He became depressed and withdrawn as his condition worsened.

In an interview with a physician and a social worker the man expressed his fear of returning to work, where he was sure that he would not survive one more accident. He was concerned about ridicule from his coworkers who, he said, blamed him for the accidents, and he was also convinced that his "disabling" symptoms would make it impossible for him to return to work. Since he was not trained for any other kind of job, and he was nearing retirement age, he feared that he would never work again.

Multiple chemical sensitivities are sometimes mistakenly diagnosed as allergies. While a person can be allergic to a certain chemical, formaldehyde as an example, he will have a reaction only to that chemical and not others. The person with multiple chemical sensitivities will have reactions to a wide range of nonrelated chemicals, whether he is also allergic to them or not.

Another psychological disturbance occurring in the workplace is a phenomenon called *mass psychogenic illness*. Similar to mass hysteria, mass psychogenic illness in the workplace results in an epidemic of many persons seemingly affected by some adverse condition that actually affected one. Such an early workplace example was recorded by Hecker in 1787, cited in "The Psychiatric Epidemic in the American Workplace."[12] He related the story of a woman putting a mouse down the blouse of a coworker—a woman with an abnormal fear of mice—who immediately went into convulsions. Her convulsions lasted for twenty-four hours and the next day three other women suffered convulsions. The following day, twenty-four women had been affected. The "cotton poisoning," as it was called, then spread to other factories in the area.

Mass psychogenic illness may be at work in some cases of poor indoor air quality, sometimes called "sick building syndrome." Low levels of irritants, combined with inadequate fresh air intake and other environmental factors such as low humidity, create a less than ideal indoor air quality. While workers exposed to this environment may be afflicted with fatigue, headaches, poor concentration, nausea, dizziness, and other symptoms, some workers will be more symptomatic than others. When these few workers complain about their symptoms, the problem comes to light and their coworkers suddenly find themselves "sick" in what appears to be a workplace epidemic.

We are not saying that all cases of poor indoor air quality are "in the head" and that symptomatic workers are imagining their complaints. We are pointing out, however, the difficulty in trying to correct indoor air quality problems to the satisfaction of all workers.

Who Is Affected?

The number of workers with the potential for exposures to psychological disorders in the workplace is likely to increase as a result of emerging trends in our economy, in technology, and in the demographics of the American workforce.

Half of the twenty fastest-growing occupations in the U.S. are in the health and computer fields, industries that have a fair amount of stress associated with them. Because of the exacting demands of their jobs, and the possibly severe consequences that can result when they fail to carry out their jobs properly, health professionals (doctors, nurses, health technologists, and dentists) have a high degree of occupational stress and other psychological disorders. They also have higher than expected rates of suicide and of alcohol or drug abuse. Nurses have increased rates of hospital and mental health center admissions for mental disorders.[13] These rates will no doubt increase as the health care sector grows.

The use of computers and robots in the workplace is increasing at a rapid pace, reducing the roles of many workers, if not eliminating them entirely. It is estimated that computers and robots will soon affect as many as 7 million factory and 38 million office jobs. Projected effects will include the loss of jobs and the addition of more lower-paying jobs, both of which can affect psychological well-being.

Jobs in the service sector have also shown a rapid rise in the last few years, a trend that shows no signs of abating. At least one study has already shown workers in the service sector to be at an increased risk of psychological disorders caused by the workplace. With the number of these jobs increasing, there is reason to believe that more workers will suffer workplace-induced psychological problems.

Other occupations that are on the rise are cashiers, waiters and waitresses, registered nurses, janitorial workers, and truck drivers. Workers in these fields often find their opportunities for growth and development to be limited. They may also find limited availability of benefits. These factors may result in increased stress and job dissatisfaction, contributing to poor mental health.

Another group of workers that must cope with stress and other psychological effects in the workplace are police and firemen. Their daily activities are filled with uncertainty, tension, and stress and the tragic events they witness over the years can exact a heavy psychological toll.

While female workers take on new roles in the workplace, in many cases they are expected to maintain their traditional roles as mothers and homemakers as well. The demands of multiple roles, combined with job dissatisfaction that large numbers of women still experience in the workplace as a result of discrimination, can ultimately lead to a rise in psychological disorders among female workers.

Any discussion of workplace psychological disorders has to take into consideration workplace violence and suicide.

Violence in the workplace has recently received considerable attention in the press because of several incidents involving disgruntled postal workers murdering coworkers; "going postal" has become a euphemism for acts of sudden, irrational violence. However, the problem of workplace violence is much more serious than these sensational, highly publicized acts of coworker violence. Bureau of Labor statistics for 1995 indicated that 20 workers are murdered and 18,000 are assaulted *each week* while on the job.[14] Taxicab drivers, convenience store clerks and other retail workers, security guards and police officers, hotel clerks, bartenders, health care workers, and social services workers are just some of the many professions that carry with them an element of risk for workplace violence.

By workplace violence we mean not only murder and assault, but also threats of assault and other violent acts such as hostage situations and rape. The circumstances of workplace violence vary and may include robbery-associated violence; violence by disgruntled clients, customers, patients, inmates, etc.; violence by coworkers, employees, or employers; and domestic violence that finds its way into the workplace.

There are several reasons why we need to treat workplace violence as separate from violence in the general population:

- Violence is a substantial contributor to death and injury on the job; NIOSH data indicates that homicide has become the second-leading cause of occupational injury death.
- The circumstances of workplace violence differ significantly from those of all other homicides. For example, 75 percent of all workplace homicides were robbery-related, compared to only 9 percent in the general population.

- Workplace violence is clustered in particular occupational settings. More than half of all workplace homicides occurred in retail trade and service industries. With the U.S. economy continuing to shift toward service sectors, workplace violence will continue to be an important occupational safety and health issue.
- Since the risk of workplace violence is associated with specific workplace factors such as dealing with the public, the exchange of money, and the delivery of services and goods, specific prevention efforts can be made to minimize the risk of violence. These may include bullet-resistant barriers in taxicabs and other areas where workers come in direct contact with the public; locked drop safes in retail establishments; and threat assessment policies in all workplaces.

There has been much discussion about the relationship between stress and violence in the workplace. The most important thing to remember is that stress can be both a cause and an effect of workplace violence. High levels of stress on the job may possibly lead to violence, but a violent incident in the workplace will almost certainly lead to stress and perhaps even to post-traumatic stress disorder.

Stress may sometimes lead to suicide in the workplace. The stress may be induced by a serious workplace injury or illness that causes the worker to become depressed and suicidal. Post-traumatic stress may also lead to suicide in the workplace.

It is difficult, however, to link a worker's suicide to the workplace, exclusive of any other factor. Sigmund Freud said that the three most important parts of a person's life are love, work, and play, and for many of us, work takes up most of our time, and in many ways defines who we are. There is no doubt that what happens to a worker on the job can have deep and lasting psychological effects, and depending upon that worker's unique psychological characteristic, can affect him in a bad way, perhaps even to the point of suicide. But since so many other factors in a person's private life affect his mental health, it is difficult, although not impossible, for workers' compensation to be paid out in the event of a worker's suicide.

A Sound Mind

How do you minimize the daily stress of your job? How can you protect yourself from an unpleasant supervisor or an act of workplace violence? Unlike other workplace diseases and injuries, there isn't a lot that you can do to protect yourself from psychological disturbances. One thing you can do, however, is make a concerted effort to reduce stress in your life. You may not be able to do too much to reduce workplace stress, but if you can eliminate stress from other areas of your life, you may find dealing with it on the job just a little easier. Your personal physician or your corporate wellness program can give you ideas on how to reduce stress, some of which may include exercise and meditation.

Reducing, modifying, or eliminating stressful situations and work practices in the workplace can go a long way toward preserving the good mental health of workers. As an example, the U.S. Postal Service, recognizing its rigid management style, has implemented two programs designed to improve quality, morale, and productivity, all of which can be adversely affected by workers with workplace-induced psychological disturbances.[15] The crew chief program provides for the local union and management to jointly select workers to act as crew chiefs, whose responsibilities are to assist the work crews in various ways, including resolving routine problems. The crew chiefs serve almost as advisers and act as something of a buffer between the crew members and supervisors.

The Postal Service's group leader program has similar goals of allowing workers to assume some supervisory duties while simultaneously allowing other workers to work with less supervision.

Corporations should analyze their workplaces to determine what conditions may lead to psychological disturbances and how they can be corrected. They should evaluate the psychological impact of shift work or night work and try to improve work schedules. Some methods are:

- Consider alternatives to permanent night shift.
- Keep consecutive night shifts to a minimum.
- Avoid quick shift changes.
- Plan some free weekends for workers on a 7-day schedule.
- Avoid several days of work followed by 4–7-day mini-vacations.
- Keep long work shifts and overtime to a minimum.
- Consider different lengths for shifts.
- Exercise at start and end times of shifts.
- Keep the schedule regular and predictable.
- Examine rest breaks as to whether there are enough of them and they are long enough.

The psychological impact of boring, repetitive tasks; of work pace and workload; and of relationships between workers and supervisors, and workers and coworkers should also be examined, all with an eye toward making whatever changes are necessary to create a mentally sound workplace.

Supervisors should be trained to identify symptoms of psychological disturbances, especially in occupations in which such disorders have been prevalent. Supervisors should be trained to take seriously any threat of violence or suicide made by a worker and should know how and when to report such threats to the appropriate officials. Even with proper identification and reporting of potential disturbances, the psychological integrity of the workplace cannot be maintained unless there is adequate, trained staff in the medical department, including psychiatrists, psychologists, and social workers with the know-how to treat affected workers, or there is some system in place to ensure that workers have access to such professionals off the job.

When it comes to protecting workers from workplace violence it is first helpful to identify risk factors on the job. These factors include the following:

- Contact with the public
- Exchange of money
- Delivery of passengers, goods, or services
- Having a mobile workplace such as a taxi or police cruiser
- Working with unstable or volatile persons in health care, social service, or criminal justice settings
- Working alone or in small numbers
- Working late at night or during early-morning hours
- Working in high-crime areas
- Guarding valuable property or possessions
- Working in community-based settings.

Once these risks are identified on a given job, the proper measures to reduce the incidence of violence can be implemented. These measures may include new environmental designs; bulletproof barriers and enclosures; counters that provide physical barriers between workers and others; locked drop safes and carrying less cash; better lighting and improved visibility; security systems; protective personal clothing; and cashless transactions in taxicabs and retail settings, using machines that accommodate automatic teller account cards or debit cards.

Administrative controls that might be implemented include changes in staffing plans and work practices to make sure that workers are not alone in vulnerable situations or that extra security is available. Policies and procedures for assessing and reporting threats should be set up. These allow employers to track and assess the potential for violence in the workplace so that it can be eliminated before it becomes a serious problem.

Worker training programs that teach employees how to react in violent situations and training in nonviolent response and conflict resolution can also help to reduce workplace violence. In addition, training that addresses specific hazards on the job and teaches prevention strategies should be included.

References

1. Camus, Albert. 1991. *The Myth of Sisyphus and Other Essays.* New York: Vintage Books.
2. National Safety Council. 1997. "Drivers Face Stress From Train Suicides." *Safety + Health* November.
3. Warshaw M.D., Leon J. 1988. "Occupational Stress." *Occupational Medicine: State of the Art Reviews* 3:4 (Philadelphia: Hanley & Belfus, Inc.).
4. McLean M.D., Alan A. 1988. "Stress Reactions in the Job Setting: Case Examples." *Occupational Medicine: State of the Art Reviews* 3:4 (Philadelphia: Hanley & Belfus, Inc.).
5. National Institute for Occupational Safety and Health (NIOSH). 1988. *Proposed National Strategies for the Prevention of Leading Work-Related Diseases and Injuries: Psychological Disorders.* Cincinnati: NIOSH.
6. Ibid.
7. Ibid.
8. Ibid.
9. Ibid.
10. Ibid.

11. Lewis, Beth M. 1987. "Workers With Multiple Chemical Sensitivities: Psychosocial Intervention." *Occupational Medicine: State of the Art Reviews* 2:4 (Philadelphia: Hanley & Belfus, Inc.).
12. Brodsky Ph.D., M.D., Carroll M. 1988. "The Psychiatric Epidemic in the American Workplace." *Occupational Medicine: State of the Art Reviews* 3:4 (Philadelphia: Hanley & Belfus, Inc.).
13. National Institute for Occupational Safety and Health (NIOSH). 1988. *Proposed National Strategies for the Prevention of Leading Work-Related Diseases and Injuries: Psychological Disorders*. Cincinnati: NIOSH.
14. National Institute for Occupational Safety and Health (NIOSH). 1996. *Violence in the Workplace: Risk Factors and Prevention Strategies*. Cincinnati: NIOSH.
15. Cabral, Roxanne. 1996. "Policies for Developing Workplace Violence Prevention Strategies." *Occupational Medicine: State of the Art Reviews* 11:2 (Philadelphia: Hanley & Belfus, Inc.).

CHAPTER 7

Heart Sick

Tony was hard at work in the basement of the old county courthouse. The contractor for which he worked was remodeling the building and Tony tackled his job with the energy and enthusiasm of a man half his age. Even at 56 years old, he still thought of himself as a young man. A lot of the guys on the crew were younger than he—could have been his grandsons—and teased the "old man," but he didn't mind. He could take a joke and he loved his job.

He was teamed up with Sam, a likable young kid, as they worked to break through some old concrete walls enclosing a closet-sized space that may once have been used as the county vault. The concrete was especially thick, so they had brought down a gasoline-powered concrete saw to help them cut through the walls. A portable space heater kept them warm in the unheated basement.

It was slow work as Tony maneuvered the saw in the tiny space. After half an hour of hard work he sat back and took a break. Sam took his turn on the saw.

A few minutes later the foremen came down to the basement and told Sam he was needed upstairs for a while.

"Look at you in there," the foreman joked with Tony, "like a monkey in a cage."

"It is kind of small, isn't it?" he said.

"Listen, Tony, take it easy while the kid's not here," the foreman said. "I'll send him back down as soon as I can."

"No problem, boss."

When the foreman had gone, Tony went back to work, attacking the old concrete with a vengeance. Progress was slow and before too long, he found himself growing tired. Maybe he was too old for this job, after all, he thought.

As the saw continued to rip at the concrete, his eyelids grew heavy and he felt himself becoming dizzy. He leaned against the wall. It was odd, he thought, that he felt so sleepy.

When Sam returned to the basement, he found Tony on the floor, slumped against the wall. His 911 call was too late.

The coroner's report indicated that Tony died from cardiac failure caused by carbon monoxide poisoning. The fumes may have come from the concrete saw, the space heater, or both and had accumulated to a lethal level in the confined space.

Cardiovascular diseases are the leading causes of disability and death in the United States. These afflictions include ischemic heart disease and hypertensive, cerebrovascular, and peripheral vascular diseases. Much has been learned about cardiovascular disease and how to control it. Most of us know that weight control, a proper diet, exercise, stress reduction, and abstaining from smoking and drinking can all help to keep us "heart healthy." We know also that age, gender, and family history play a part in the incidence of cardiovascular disease. What we are only now beginning to understand is to what extent workplace factors can be linked to cardiovascular diseases, either as causative agents or as agents that can make a bad situation worse.

Coronary heart disease, hypertension, and related diseases have a high incidence among the general population in the U.S., and so are frequently found in workers who may find their conditions exacerbated by workplace factors. Other diseases, such as arrhythmias (irregular heartbeat) and cardiomyopathies (diseases of heart muscle), are more directly related to specific occupational exposures or conditions. Exposures to workplace hazards, such as carbon monoxide in the case of Tony, can have an immediate and fatal effect upon the heart, regardless of whether or not a prior cardiovascular disease was present.

The Problem

The numbers are not definite, but existing information on the relationship between workplace factors and cardiovascular disease indicates that millions of workers are currently exposed to work-related factors that can be linked to an increased risk of cardiovascular disease. These factors are of two types; the first includes exposures to workplace agents that actually induce or aggravate a physical disorder. The second type includes psychosocial factors in the workplace that may have an adverse effect on the cardiovascular system.

The National Institute for Occupational Safety and Health (NIOSH) Registry of Toxic Effects of Chemical Substances lists 1,466 chemicals as having possible cardiotoxic effects.[1] A few common agents from the list are carbon disulfide, which can result in chronic cardiovascular disease; carbon monoxide, which can cause heart failure and immediate death; halogenated hydrocarbons, responsible for acute arrhythmias; and nitroglycerin and related compounds. Occupational exposures to antimony, cadmium, cobalt, and lead have also been shown to increase the risk of cardiovascular disease.

Carbon monoxide poisoning is a problem that exists in many different work sites, although the severity will vary depending upon the extent of exposure to the gas, and other environmental and physical conditions. Carbon monoxide readily combines with hemoglobin, the molecule in red blood cells responsible for bringing oxygen to the body's organs and tissues. The new molecule, carboxyhemoglobin, has less oxygen-carrying capacity so that organs such as the heart receive less oxygen and are therefore unable to perform at their full potential. Some studies have shown that carbon monoxide exposure increases the risk of cardiovascular morbidity and mortality, and in persons with underlying coronary heart disease, carbon monoxide poisoning may cause angina, cardiac arrhythmia, acute myocardial infarction, or sudden death.[2]

The use of gasoline-powered engines that release carbon monoxide is a particular health problem. A study of several car carrier ships found that workers who off-load the cars are routinely exposed to carbon monoxide levels inside the ships that exceed the Occupational Safety and Health Administration's (OSHA) ceiling limit of 200 ppm (a ceiling limit means that at no time should the concentration of the chemical in question exceed the established limit; in this case, 200 ppm).[3] Workers at indoor skating arenas who use gasoline-powered resurfacing machines are at risk of carbon monoxide exposures as a result of engine exhaust. In one Seattle ice arena, carbon monoxide levels reached 354 ppm and 78 people were sent to emergency rooms with symptoms of fatigue, dizziness, headache, and acute respiratory distress.[4]

A slightly different study of an indoor sports arena in Quebec City, Canada, also showed unsafe levels of carbon monoxide from engine exhaust during an indoor motocross competition.[5] The protocol of the 1994 study called for an officer from the Centre de Sante Publique de Quebec to halt the proceedings if the level of carbon monoxide exceeded 50 ppm (the occupational standard used by the province of Quebec), until such time as the levels fell below the standard. The competition was interrupted seven times for intervals ranging from 4 to 12 minutes each because the carbon monoxide standard was exceeded. Even though the arena was equipped with a high-performance ventilation system that generally prevented toxic levels of carbon monoxide from occurring, minor peaks above the standard did occur. It is entirely possible that a serious health problem could have occurred in an arena with a less efficient ventilation system. This study also pointed out the importance of monitoring for carbon monoxide in closed or poorly ventilated areas in which gasoline-powered engines or other equipment are in use.

The construction industry frequently uses gasoline-powered tools and equipment on job sites because of their portability and efficiency and because of the scarcity of electricity. Troweling machines, saws, mixers, and small-wheeled loaders are examples of carbon monoxide–generating equipment that are often used in confined spaces, thereby creating a health risk for workers. In 1993, at a building under construction in Ontario, Canada, one worker died from cardiac failure and six more were hospitalized when a gasoline-powered trowel machine and a gasoline-powered cement mixer were operated simultaneously with two propane-powered forklifts.[6]

The incidence of cardiovascular disease among Finnish foundry workers exposed to carbon monoxide was investigated by researchers from the Institute of Occupational Health, Helsinki, and the Department of General Practice and Primary Health Care at the University of Helsinki, Finland.[7] While carbon monoxide exposures at high levels can lead to immediate heart failure, lower exposures over time also can have adverse effects upon the cardiovascular system. The 1987 study was designed to examine these long-term effects and reviewed the medical records of 2,857 men hired between 1950 and 1972 by 20 Finnish foundries. The results showed that long-term occupational exposures to carbon monoxide increased the risk of cardiovascular morbidity (incidence of disease) and mortality. Since carbon monoxide in the circulatory system will replace oxygen in blood hemoglobin, the net effect is reduced oxygen delivery to the heart. The Finnish study showed an increased risk of cardiovascular disease among workers who already had a reduced capacity to deliver oxygen to the heart, as in smokers.

Excessive carbon monoxide levels have also been demonstrated among warehouse and materials handling workers who use propane-powered forklifts indoors[8] and among janitorial workers using propane-powered floor burnishers.[9]

In addition to chemical agents, other workplace conditions such as heatstroke and noise have been shown to be associated with cardiovascular disease, with heatstroke having the potential for an immediate lethal effect. Some studies performed in Europe and South America showed evidence that workers employed for a prolonged time in a hot industry have a higher morbidity rate from cardiovascular disease than other workers.[10] As record high temperatures are seemingly being set every summer, heat stroke becomes a very real threat to many workers.

Excessive physical exertion in a hot environment can result in heatstroke; the heart and circulatory system are simply unable to meet the demands placed upon them by exertion and the rigors of the environment. Early signs and symptoms of heatstroke may include dizziness, nausea, and severe headache. Strange as it may seem, a heatstroke victim stops sweating. His skin becomes dry and hot and he will run a body temperature as high as 106°F and climbing. In addition, a worker suffering from heatstroke will demonstrate odd behavior, characterized by confusion, delirium, and coma. The circulatory system may be affected, causing the person to go into shock. If cooling of the stricken worker's body does not begin immediately, irreversible damage to vital organs may develop, leading to death.

There are some steps recommended by NIOSH that companies can follow to minimize the risk of heatstroke for their workers.

- Establish criteria for a heat alert; one should be declared if the temperature for the next day is predicted to be 95°F or higher or a maximum of 90°F if the predicted maximum is 9°F above the maximum reached in any of the preceding three days; this formula takes into account a worker gradually becoming acclimatized to the heat.
- Postpone tasks that are not urgent until the hot spell is over.
- Increase rest allowances; let workers recover in air-conditioned places.
- Turn off unnecessary heat sources such as equipment that may not be needed at that time.
- Remind workers to drink water in small amounts frequently to prevent excessive dehydration; workers should weigh themselves before and after their shifts and drink enough water to maintain body weight.
- Monitor the environmental heat at the job site and resting places.
- Check workers' oral temperatures during their most severe exposure period.
- Exercise additional caution on the first day of a shift

change to make sure that workers are not overexposed to heat, because they may have lost some of their acclimatization over the weekend and during days off.

- Send any worker who exhibits even minor signs of a heat disorder to the medical officer; the worker should not return to work without the physician's written permission.
- Restrict overtime work.

The psychosocial factors in the workplace that may lead to cardiovascular disease are discussed in length in Chapter Six and so will not be repeated here. It is enough to say that occupational stress frequently leads to hypertension (high blood pressure), which may, of course, lead to more serious cardiovascular diseases.

Who Is at Risk?

Are there certain occupations that have a higher risk of cardiovascular disease than others? Most of us would probably agree that we suffer at least some occasional stress on the job, but in the majority of cases, these minor episodes are not life threatening. There are some occupations, however, in which stress is experienced so often it almost becomes a part of the job description. These stressful jobs could result in cardiovascular disease. When these stress-causing conditions are combined with cardiotoxic chemicals and physical agents in the workplace, there is an even greater risk of disease.

Truck, taxi, and bus drivers are examples of workers who fall into this category; they are exposed to stress, as well as chemical and physical agents that can cause cardiovascular disease. Studies performed by the Institute of Environmental Medicine at the Karolinska Institute in Sweden in the 1970s and '80s examined the causes of death and the risks of developing myocardial infarction (a condition characterized by areas of dead heart muscle) among urban bus drivers.[11] In the mortality study, 9,446 male bus drivers in two Swedish counties that contained major urban areas (Stockholm and Goteborg) were found to have had a 50-60 percent increased mortality from myocardial infarction, compared to other employed men in these counties. A second study demonstrated a 60 percent increased incidence of myocardial infarction for bus drivers in Stockholm County, compared to men employed in other work in the county. A third study examined bus drivers employed by Stockholm Transport in the 1970s and found that death from, as well as incidence of, myocardial infarction was elevated for bus drivers at the company, compared to other men in Stockholm County. The risks were greater for middle-aged drivers, between 55 and 64 years of age, who showed mortality from myocardial infarction at rates twice as high as their counterparts working in other occupations.

These studies determined that there were several factors that could have caused the increased incidence of myocardial infarctions among bus drivers. The researchers took into consideration lifestyle differences such as smoking and dietary habits but concluded that workplace factors such as stress, irregular working hours, noise, and emissions from automobile exhaust played an important part in the development of the disease among the drivers.

In a 1986–1988 German study, researchers from the Department of Occupational Medicine at Volkswagen AG and from the Institute of Clinical Chemistry in Munich examined risk factors for the incidence of myocardial infarction among 65 workers.[12] The study focused on two workplace factors, shift work and exposures to noise. While the researchers did not find that noise contributed to the development of myocardial infarctions, they did find that it may be a risk factor for hypertension, which could lead to heart disease. They also found that shift work, most notably night work, may act as a risk factor for myocardial infarctions, especially when combined with smoking.

Both the Swedish and German studies showed an increased risk of cardiovascular disease (myocardial infarction) as a result of both psychosocial and chemical/physical agents in the workplace.

Clerical workers and firefighters are two other groups that have been shown to have a greater risk of cardiovascular disease with causes grounded in the workplace. For clerical workers, the precipitating causes are centered around occupational stress, which leads to hypertension and various cardiovascular diseases.

Heart disease has long been recognized as a significant health risk for firefighters. The problem is so prevalent that 36 states have some type of heart presumption disability law on the books for firefighters. In addition to occupational stress, firefighters are also routinely exposed to a wide range of chemical and physical agents that may, by themselves, lead to cardiovascular disease. Carbon monoxide and cyanide, in particular, are known cardiac toxicants to which firefighters are routinely exposed (cyanide exposure is low in most fires but may be elevated in fires in which certain types of plastic are burning). In addition to these toxicants, firefighters also experience exposures to particulates in the smoke, acrolein, hydrogen chloride, nitrogen dioxide, polynuclear aromatic compounds, and benzene, all of which are respiratory irritants that may affect pulmonary function. These short-term decreases in pulmonary function, in turn, create a demand on the cardiovascular system that may result in heart disease.

It is not always easy to determine the role cardiovascular disease plays as a factor contributing to mortality among firemen. Part of this difficulty lies in the "healthy worker effect." Certain occupations, such as fire fighting and police work, require a degree of physical fitness that generally exceeds that of workers in the general population. Workers in these physically demanding occupations may be considered more healthy than others and may have a lower mortality rate in general. When groups of firefighters or other "healthy" workers are compared to workers in other occupations, a significantly lower mortality rate due to cardiovascular disease is seen among the firefighters. In order to determine an accurate rate of cardiovascular disease among such workers, researchers must then compensate for the healthy worker effect.

It is also important to remember that mortality studies, by their very nature, examine only cardiovascular disease deaths and do not tell us anything about the incidence of significant heart disease, such as myocardial infarction, among firefighters.

In almost any occupation, it is difficult to attribute workplace factors to the existence of cardiovascular disease in any given individual. Such variables as age, weight, activity level, family history, smoking and drinking, and diet confuse the picture and may mask the disease's workplace origin or the additive effects caused by workplace conditions. No one is surprised if an overweight, out-of-shape, 65-year-old, smoking, drinking, junk-food eating male drops dead from a heart attack. He brought it upon himself, we may say. Yet, that may not be entirely true. No doubt his lifestyle and physical condition set him up for a heart attack, but can we be certain that exposures to workplace chemicals didn't gradually destroy the muscles of his heart, making him more vulnerable to a heart attack? Do we know for sure how much his hypertension was caused by occupational stress as compared to smoking, drinking, and obesity? An autopsy may reveal an enlarged heart, blocked arteries, or damaged heart muscle, but none of those physical findings would make the case for a heart attack caused by occupational factors rather than lifestyle factors, or vice versa. We simply wouldn't know.

These questions have created an interesting debate in the area of workers' compensation claims arising from fatal heart attacks. It has caused the families of retired California firemen and policemen to file claims for fatal heart attacks incurred by their loved ones *after* retirement on the grounds that their heart conditions were brought on by occupational factors.

In a slightly different case, the family of a man who died of a massive heart attack while rushing to help another worker injured on the job filed a claim for compensation.[13] The claim was contested by the company and four years later the case wound up in the Supreme Court. The court agreed that workers' compensation should only be paid if the injury or death rises out of and is in the course of the worker's employment. The first part, "out of," questions where the accident happened. In this case, the deceased worker was at a job site. The second part, "in the course of," refers to whether the worker was doing work-related activities at the time of the injury. Here, the Supreme Court found that in addition to duties specified in the worker's job description, there might be other, unspecified duties that would constitute "work," and that responding to emergencies was one of them. The family won their case and was awarded workers' compensation.

Whether the claim is for heart attack or some other occupational disease or injury, there are some problems inherent in workers' compensation that are worth discussing here.

The first problem is that there is no uniformity in workers' compensation statutes. Each state enacts its own statutes and no two states have exactly the same laws. This results in a hodgepodge of workers' compensation laws in which a worker in one state might receive compensation for a knee injury, let's say, but be ineligible for compensation in a neighboring state. Some states disallow compensation if there were preexisting injuries, while others do not. The various states have different definitions of what constitutes a work site, meaning you may or may not be compensated for an injury in your employer's parking lot or on the way to or from work, depending on your state's laws.

This confusing condition also creates a nightmare for businesses. Since the states all set different rates that businesses must pay for workers' compensation, a business paying high rates to a state with liberal compensation may be at a competitive disadvantage to an out-of-state business that does not pay as much. If a business operates in more than one state, it is subject to several sets of workers' compensation statutes and several different sets of rates. This means that the company spends a lot of money on legal and administrative matters and wastes a lot of time handling claims.

Another problem with workers' compensation is that it is a monopoly within any state. There is only one system for handling claims, and compensation rates are usually set by the state legislature. Without competition, there is no incentive to reduce administrative costs or to make the system more efficient.

Compensation disputes and interpretations of workers' compensation statutes are usually the responsibility of a special administrative court set up for those purposes. Lawyers who serve in these courts are specialists in administrative or labor laws. The problem with this system is that the lawyers who are appointed to these courts tend to be biased toward either labor or business, or are politically motivated, thereby resulting in legal decisions that may have less to do with the merits of the case than they do with other extenuating circumstances. Another problem with this court system is that it is very inefficient. Because one state's workers' compensation statutes have no bearing on those of another state, lawyers cannot cite precedence from a case in Vermont, as an example, to be used in a case in Oklahoma. Lawyers must start from scratch in each case, a method that wastes both time and money.

The way in which a work-relation is established between injury and the job is another problem for the workers' compensation system. As discussed earlier, it is sometimes difficult to establish a direct cause and effect between an injury and the workplace, and the picture becomes even more confused by the states' various interpretations of "workplace." In the Supreme Court example above we spoke about injury or death that "rises out of and is in the course of the worker's employment." What happens when a state changes the word "and" to "or"? Now, there is less to prove in order to substantiate a claim and some might say that there is an increased risk of false claims being filed.

The problem with the work-relation principle is that it *does* make it easier for an unscrupulous, or well-intentioned but mistaken, worker to file a workers' compensation claim simply by claiming his injury, whatever it may be, was caused by a workplace event. The weekend warrior who strains his back in a pickup basketball game on Sunday can come into work on Monday and claim he injured his back on the job last Friday. Who can prove that didn't happen? The burden of proof is always on the company to prove that the injury was not work-related.

Let's understand something here. There are angels and devils on both sides. There are "workers" who travel from state to state filing false workers' compensation claims as a way of life and there are unconscionable companies that fight every claim brought against them, no matter how clear-cut they may seem. On the other hand, there are workers who honestly believe their injuries are work-related, even though they may not be able to pinpoint the exact date or cause of the injury, just as there are companies that take their responsibilities to their employees seriously and pay legitimate claims (and sometimes illegitimate claims that cannot be conclusively disproved).

It is obvious that the present system of workers' compensation has its shortcomings, inefficiencies, and abuses. It is time we started asking ourselves what we expect and need from such a system.

Heart Healthy

Because we don't know exactly to what extent workplace conditions may affect the cardiovascular system is all the more reason to try to reduce, if not eliminate, these conditions. Cardiovascular disease is a health problem well-known to the general public. Health care practitioners and various public and private agencies have been vocal about ways to prevent cardiovascular disease; the same energy should be expended in the workplace, where disease factors are so prevalent.

As a general rule, programs that advocate health promotion and disease prevention should be set up in the workplace wherever possible. There is some movement toward this goal already, with companies establishing wellness programs that may include access to health clubs, in addition to workplace educational programs. The workplace affords a great opportunity for health care practitioners to educate a great number of people about the risks of cardiovascular disease. In an ideal situation, both environmental and personal risks would be addressed through appropriate strategies in the workplace. In workplaces with no identifiable chemical or physical agent posing a cardiovascular risk, the program would focus on strategies that would help workers stop smoking, reduce stress, improve their diet and exercise regimen, and generally help them shape a new, more healthful lifestyle, one that would reduce their chances of developing cardiovascular disease.

In the workplace reducing the effects of chemical/physical agents that can cause cardiovascular disease is a necessary step toward creating a "heart healthy" environment. As always, better hazards communications and a better understanding of workplace cardiotoxins help to ensure workers' health. Companies that comply with current exposure criteria or develop and install better control technology can significantly reduce the risks of occupational cardiovascular disease. Better environmental control programs, such as an effective protocol for working in confined spaces, as well as workplace and medical monitoring, can also add to the margin of safety. Also, companies must be willing to implement new or improved standards as they are developed and should take the lead in identifying and controlling new industrial exposures to cardiotoxic agents.

Of course, the best thing you can do to protect yourself from cardiovascular disease in the workplace is to keep yourself in top physical condition. You've heard it all before—proper diet, exercise, stress reduction, abstinence from smoking and alcohol—but it makes sense. Keeping yourself "heart healthy" at home will protect you at work as well.

References

1. National Institute for Occupational Safety and Health (NIOSH). 1986. *Proposed National Strategies for the Prevention of Leading Work-Related Diseases and Injuries: Occupational Cardiovascular Diseases*. Cincinnati: NIOSH.
2. Haflidson, William O. 1997. "Carbon Monoxide Exposure of Concrete Finishers." *Applied Occupational and Environmental Hygiene* 12:2.
3. Davenport, Aaron C. and William C. Hinds. 1996. "Carbon Monoxide and Oxides of Nitrogen During Off-loading of Car Carrier Vessels." *Applied Occupational and Environmental Hygiene* 11:12.
4. McNabb, Nigel, Jeff Kostiuk and Michael Brauer. 1997. "Improved Ice Arena Air Quality With the Use of a Three-Way Catalytic Converter and Fuel Management System." *AIHA Journal* 58:8.
5. Levesque, Benoit et al. 1997. "Indoor Motocross Competitions: Air Quality Evaluation." *AIHA Journal* 58:4.
6. Haflidson, William O. 1997. "Carbon Monoxide Exposure of Concrete Finishers." *Applied Occupational and Environmental Hygiene* 12:2.
7. Koskela, R., M. Klockars and E. Jarvinen. 1992. "Cardiovascular Diseases Among Foundry Workers Exposed to Carbon Monoxide." *Proceedings of the 9th. International Symposium on Epidemiology in Occupational Health*. Cincinnati: NIOSH.
8. McCammon, Jane B., Lyle E. McKenzie and Michele Heinzman. 1996. "Carbon Monoxide Poisoning Related to the Indoor Use of Propane-Fueled Forklifts in Colorado Workplaces." *Applied Occupational and Environmental Hygiene* 11:3.
9. Demer, Frank R., Julia C. Rosen and Timothy J. Finman. 1996. "Carbon Monoxide Exposures During the Use of Propane-Powered Floor Burnishers." *Applied Occupational and Environmental Hygiene* 11:8.
10. National Institute for Occupational Safety and Health

(NIOSH). 1977. *Occupational Diseases: A Guide to Their Recognition*. Cincinnati: NIOSH.

11. Alfredsson, L., N. Hammar and C. Hogstedt. 1992. "Increased Risk of Myocardial Infarction Among Bus Drivers in Urban Areas." *Proceedings of the 9th. International Symposium on Epidemiology in Occupational Health*. Cincinnati: NIOSH.
12. Ibid.
13. Pierce, F. David. 1996. *Shifting Safety and Health Paradigms*. Rockville: Government Institutes, Inc.

CHAPTER 8

Why Johnny Can't Hear

The filling and packaging machinery of the hand lotion company filled a building as long as a football field. When all the machines were up and running, it was almost impossible for two people to hear each other over the noise.

It was not quite as loud where Shirley operated the bottle-capping machine. She had been responsible for that piece of machinery for the last three years and had come to know its whims and peculiarities as well as she knew her children's. It was an antiquated piece of equipment, due to be replaced in the next year, and she could tell how well the machine was operating just from its sound. She knew that when she heard a slight rasping noise coming from it, like fingernails on coarse sandpaper, it was low on oil and in danger of overheating. It was not always easy to hear the sound, but so far she had been able to catch it and add oil in time to keep the machine running. If the machine overheated, it would shut down the entire packaging line.

Shirley was proud of her work, and so the first time she missed the telltale sounds of the overheated machine and it ground to a halt, shutting down the line for two hours, she was embarrassed and angry with herself. The foreman was irritated by the accident, but considering

Shirley's years of good work habits, he was not as hard on her as she was on herself.

A week later the machine overheated again and the line shut down. This time the old machine was damaged and had to be repaired, a costly proposition, especially when the company had hoped to keep the machine going until it could be replaced.

Shirley was nervous as she sat across from the foreman in his office. She didn't know what was happening to her. Two shutdowns in two weeks; it wasn't like her.

"I don't understand it," the foreman said, "you've always been one of the best workers on the floor, and now this. What's going on?"

"I don't know," she said. "I can't seem to tell anymore when it's starting to heat up. I just can't hear it."

The foreman nodded. "I'm no doctor, but maybe you need to have your hearing checked. I like you, Shirley, but we can't afford to let this happen again."

She knew exactly what he meant. She needed this job. Maybe it was time to see a doctor.

Although anyone can experience hearing loss caused by noise, workers exposed to high levels of industrial noise show greater noise-induced hearing loss than the general population. Loss of hearing is a severe impairment in itself, but sometimes, as in Shirley's case, it can lead to other, seemingly unrelated problems.

In testimony given before the Government Regulation Subcommittee of the Senate Small Business Committee in 1975, Dr. John F. Finklea, then National Institute for Occupational Safety and Health (NIOSH) Director, said, "Workplace noise exposures, especially those occurring in mechanized industries, are likely to be the most intense and prolonged of any experienced in daily living. Because of their increased severity, occupational noise exposures can be considered as posing a greater threat to one's health and well-being than general environmental noise."[1]

Hearing loss in the workplace is not a new phenomenon and historical records documenting this health problem go back at least two hundred years. In 1713, Bernardino Ramazzini published *De Morbis Artificum Diatriba*, in which he commented on copper workers who had suffered hearing loss as a result of hammering on metal. An article in an 1830 edition of the British medical journal *Lancet* described blacksmiths' deafness from continued exposure to noise. Also in the 1800s, Thomas Barr documented noise-induced hearing loss among British boilermakers.

The Problem

While no comprehensive epidemiologic data on noise-induced hearing loss exists, the Occupational Safety and Health Administration (OSHA) estimates that at least 3 million workers in the United States are exposed to potentially hazardous daily levels of occupational noise at levels of 85 dBA (a unit of sound measurement which measures decibels adjusted to the frequency of sounds that can be heard by the human ear) and higher; at least 1.5 million workers in manufacturing have sustained job-related hearing impairment.[2] The OSHA noise standard sets a maximum exposure level of 90 dBA over an eight-hour time-weighted average (TWA), although National Institute for Occupational Safety and Health (NIOSH) recommends 85 dBA. However, the OSHA standard mandates that a hearing conservation program be established in workplaces where workers have noise exposures above 85 dBA TWA.

Here are some examples that may help you better understand dBA levels. A "quiet" room is about 40 dBA, normal conversation and a window air-conditioning unit

25 feet away are about 60 dBA. A vacuum cleaner is 70 dBA; a garbage disposal, 80 dBA; and a power lawn mower, about 95 dBA. A rock 'n' roll band pumps up the jam at about 110 dBA. As you can see by these examples, the OSHA noise standard permits you to be exposed to noise levels somewhere between a garbage disposal and a power mower. Even if you didn't experience any hearing loss, there is a good possibility that you would be irritated and put in a foul mood by all that noise.

One in four U.S. workers exposed to occupational noise levels of 90 dBA over a working lifetime will develop a hearing impairment.[3] Occupational hearing loss is a big problem and workers' compensation claims show just how big—$800 million paid out in claims from 1977 to 1987.

While loss of hearing may result from a single exposure to a very brief impulse noise or explosion, these types of loss are rare. In most cases, noise-induced hearing loss usually develops slowly and goes unnoticed in its early stages. It begins with the progressive destruction of sensory cells in the cochlea of the ear. Once these sensory cells are damaged, they are incapable of repairing themselves, nor can they be restored through medical intervention. This means that this type of hearing loss is irreversible and increases in severity with continued exposure to noise.

Hearing capability is tested by subjecting the worker to pure tones (like those produced from a tuning fork) at different frequencies and loudness. The results are recorded on an audiogram. If the worker becomes hearing impaired as a result of noise-induced hearing loss, subsequent tests will show that he will only be able to hear higher frequency sounds when they are much louder than his previous audiogram. However, the audiogram employs a pure tone at each frequency to test hearing, which is not consistent with the real world. In the workplace, industrial noise occurs over a wide range of frequencies, making up complex sounds. The hearing-impaired worker may hear the same *volume* as before but will not hear certain *frequencies* of sound as well. This would be like listening to Beethoven played by a full symphony orchestra, then hearing the same piece again with certain notes missing—there will be a big difference in what we hear between the two.

Before an individual can be shown to be impaired by noise-induced hearing loss, it is necessary to rule out all other possible causative factors. Disease, mechanical injury, and drug use are factors that can affect hearing. Also, a loss of hearing acuity is part of the natural aging process. There is a wide variance in sensitivity to hearing loss among individuals and there is some evidence to suggest that age, general health, and heredity may play a part in determining how likely a person is to experience hearing loss. In other words, some people may be predisposed toward hearing loss and workplace noise could increase their risks of such a loss. A study from Finland conducted by the Finnish Institute of Occupational Health suggests that hearing loss is aggravated, as the exposure to noise continues, in workers who have elevated cholesterol and blood pressure levels, and in the course of aging and increased exposure to noise.[4] While not completely understood, it is thought that this hearing loss may be due to decreased metabolic functions in the inner ear and disturbances in peripheral blood circulation.

Once a person is diagnosed as suffering from noise-induced hearing loss, he should be aware that other problems associated with hearing loss may beset him.

Communication often becomes a problem as a result of hearing loss in higher frequencies. Normal speech patterns of the human voice encompass various frequencies so the hearing-impaired worker will not clearly hear what someone says to him. It might sound to him like static on a radio; certain words or sounds may drop out. The worker most likely will not recognize that he has suffered a hearing loss. It will seem to him that people are mumbling and just not speaking clearly.

In addition to the obvious impairment one suffers with hearing loss, social handicaps may result, especially if the faculty of speech is affected. Anxiety, miscommunication, lowered self-esteem, and self-imposed withdrawal from society are all possible consequences of hearing loss.

The job-related consequences of hearing loss may threaten a worker's employment status, as in the case of Shirley at the beginning of this chapter. Compared to other workers, a hearing-impaired worker is at a distinct disadvantage in a noisy workplace. He may not be able to communicate effectively, especially when the job requires wearing hearing protectors. He may be unable to monitor changes in machinery sounds and he may have reduced audibility of potential safety hazards. Unfortunately, since noise-induced hearing loss is not usually discovered in the early stages, it may appear to an employer or supervisor that the worker's job performance is inexplicably deteriorating, which could result in the worker being transferred to some other job or perhaps fired.

To list here all the occupations in which noise may be a serious health risk would be impossible. Instead, let's look at a few selected occupations that will serve to exemplify the problem of hearing loss on the job.

Since 1980, NIOSH has been studying hearing loss among firefighters and EMS personnel. Firefighters are subjected daily to sirens, air horns, and the roar of diesel motors. As if noise from the equipment weren't bad enough, the construction of most fire stations does little to abate noise; shiny, hard-surfaced materials reflect sound rather than mute it. Firefighters in stations that are responsible for airport protection also have to deal with the additional noise of airplane landings and takeoffs.

Hearing loss in firefighters may result in a life-or-death situation for themselves as well as others. In smoke-filled buildings, where the visibility may be near zero, firefighters often rely on their hearing to locate persons trapped in the fire, honing in on their cries or moans. They must also listen and respond to radio communications and must be able to hear the warning sounds from an air horn signaling them to leave a building because of imminent danger.

There have been several studies of fire departments throughout the country—Los Angeles; Newburgh, NY; Pittsburgh; Hamilton, OH—all of which showed a significantly earlier onset of hearing loss among firefighters compared to the general population.[5]

New designs in fire apparatus and equipment are helping to reduce occupational noise exposures for firemen. Many vehicles now provide fully enclosed cabs for firefighters. These reduce siren, engine, and road noises. The placement of sirens and air horns upon vehicles can also affect the amount of noise reaching the firefighters onboard. Generally speaking, the more the vehicle's body can act as a shield between the siren and the firefighters, the more the noise will be reduced. Many vehicles now have the siren or air horn mounted under the front bumper or in an opening in the grille, placements that can significantly reduce the level of noise reaching the firemen.

Workers in the construction industry are also at serious risk of occupational hearing loss. The 1988 National Occupational Exposure Survey conducted by OSHA found that as many as 500,000 construction workers nationwide are routinely exposed to noise levels of 85 dBA (as an eight-hour time-weighted average) or greater while on the job.[6] Construction sites pose problems for researchers trying to study the effects of noise on workers. For one, workers share a job site with other trades and so are subjected not only to noise from their own equipment, but also from the equipment of other trades as well. Because construction noise is more often sudden and intermittent, rather than constant, it is difficult to use traditional methods of audiometry to measure workers' exposures to noise. Also, because many construction workers are self-employed, they have a high rate of mobility, moving from one job site to another, often in the same day. This makes accurate exposures to noise difficult to determine.

A study of four hundred carpenters, plumbers/pipe fitters, and heavy equipment operators in the Midwest analyzed their use of hearing protection devices and their perceptions of hearing loss on the job.[7] The study found that 44 to 65 percent of the workers reported experiencing hearing loss on the job. Yet, these workers used hearing protection devices from only 18 to 49 percent of the time they should have been used (the criteria used for the "right time" to wear hearing protection was if workers three feet away from each other, or less, had to shout to be heard over the noise). Some of the reasons advanced for their lack of hearing protection were inadequate training in when to use such devices and the use of improper hearing protection (not all hearing protection devices are the same, as they are available in an array of styles, each with different features designed for different noise-blocking functions). This study pointed out the need for mandatory hearing conservation programs for *all* construction workers, not just workers in industrial work sites who are required to have such programs.

An obvious group of workers who are exposed to

excessive noise, although they probably would not call it that, are musicians. Musicians do not often perceive excessive noise exposures as a problem. Still, with performances of one to two hours and practice times lasting several hours at any one time, musicians as a group may have a potential for hearing loss that surpasses the general public. Remember, it is higher frequencies that are lost in hearing impairment, frequencies that are especially important for musicians to be able to hear.

A 1996 study by the University of Kentucky Medical Center, Department of Preventive Medicine, in Lexington, Kentucky, was undertaken to determine the noise exposures of musicians at practice.[8] Researchers studied musicians in seven different types of musical ensembles, including a large and small high school marching band, a university marching band, a pep band, a percussion ensemble, and a six-piece soft rock band. Five noise meters were used in each monitoring session, each group having a meter microphone attached to the musicians' shoulders, slightly below ear level.

The study showed that most of the measured noise levels exceeded OSHA's permissible exposure limit, which means that a hearing conservation program would be necessary. It is estimated that the OSHA noise standard protects from 80 to 90 percent of the working population, based upon speech frequencies and not higher frequencies. This study estimated that as many as 20 percent of the musicians would lose a measurable part of their hearing acuity after a working lifetime of thirty years.

The researchers suggested the use of sound-dampening materials on walls and ceilings and heavy carpeting on the floor in practice areas to help reduce reverberation. They also recommended the use of commercially available hearing protection devices that attenuate the sound without losing any frequencies.

Noise-induced hearing loss is also a common workplace hazard among developing countries that have few, if any, occupational safety and health regulations and are often using obsolete machinery dumped there by the developed nations. A recent study conducted by the Institute of Occupational Medicine of China and the National Coal Corporation, Beijing, examined 1,502 underground coal miners exposed to occupational noise and compared them to a control group of 130 workers who were never exposed to occupational noise.[9] While the researchers found varying degrees of hearing impairment among the miners, dependent upon specific job tasks, the general incidence of hearing damage was a remarkable 48.2 percent, compared to the control group at 1.54 percent. Over 2 million miners work in Chinese mines and the majority of these mines have not adopted noise-control measures, so the potential for hearing loss remains high among these workers.

Nigeria is another developing country without strict occupational safety and health standards. As part of a continuing assessment of the impact of industrialization on Nigerian workers, researchers from the Department of Community Health at the University of Lagos' College of Medicine conducted a study of iron and steel workers.[10] These workers, employed at various tasks throughout the factory, were subjected to occupational noise levels between 66 and 120 dBA during the course of their working day. No protective hearing equipment was available to them. The study was conducted to determine if there were differences in the hearing threshold level (the level, in decibels, at which a certain frequency is detected) among the workers. The results showed that 90 of the 132 subjects working in the factory's electrical furnace and rolling mill areas had significant hearing loss in the higher frequencies. Nigeria is making progress in controlling traditional diseases among the general population, and this study suggested that urgent measures be taken in the workplace to protect the health of workers and to ensure that overall health gains are not eroded.

Although we have been discussing noise-induced hearing loss, there is also data that shows hearing impairment caused by exposures to a variety of chemicals. Pharmaceuticals, particularly aminoglycoside and other antibiotics, some diuretics, and some analgesics and antineoplastic drugs, have demonstrated ear toxicity. The same effect can occur with exposures to inorganic arsenic, mercury, carbon monoxide, carbon disulfide, organotin compounds, and organic solvents.

Loud and Clear

Unlike occupational diseases caused by exposures to chemical and even some physical agents, the causes of noise-induced hearing loss are obvious. The emphasis on protecting workers, therefore, does not need to be focused as much on investigation as it does on prevention.

There are some things you can do to protect your hearing in the workplace. You should wear whatever hearing protectors are recommended for your job and wear them properly. Too often workers refuse to wear hearing protectors because they can't get them to fit comfortably or because they fear protectors will limit their ability to perform their jobs properly or hear warning signals. The latter belief may be understandable, especially in industries where the employer has made no effort to reduce noise levels in the workplace, but it is shortsighted, considering the potential for severe hearing loss. It is important, also, that you have the right type of hearing-protection devices for your job. There are earmuffs, earplugs, and ear canal caps, all of which come in several varieties, and certain helmets that may function additionally as hearing protectors. You should know which is the right type of protection for you. Hearing protectors have ratings that will tell you, in decibels, how much noise they will reduce. Knowing the noise level of your workplace beforehand, you can select the proper hearing protector for your job.

Another way to protect your hearing in a noisy workplace is to have it tested often. Some companies may have a hearing conservation program in place that already includes regular testing. It is important to know if your company has such a program, and, if so, to make sure it is in effect and you are regularly tested. A good rule of thumb is this: If you have to shout at a coworker from an arm's length away for him to hear you, there should be a hearing conservation program set up. If your company does not have a program, you might consider having your hearing tested by your own physician.

A complete hearing conservation program will include the following elements:

- periodic noise measurements
- engineering or administrative controls to reduce excessive noise exposures
- personal ear protection
- audiometric monitoring of exposed workers.

You can also ask to be transferred to another department, or to be assigned to another task in which you will not be exposed to excessive noise. However, you should not be forced to give up a particular job because of unsafe noise levels; it is still the company's responsibility to provide a safe and healthy workplace for its employees.

Companies can aggressively act to protect the hearing of their employees by strictly enforcing the wearing of hearing protection equipment where appropriate. They also need to take responsibility for reducing workplace noise through engineering controls. This could include modification of existing machinery or the purchase of new, quieter machinery. Even the purchasing department can have an influence on noise in the workplace by making noise reduction part of its purchasing criteria; buying quieter equipment and machinery may also encourage manufacturers to develop quieter products. Supervisors can exert administrative controls to reduce workers' exposures to noise. Scheduling workers to quieter tasks in between noisy ones can help reduce their overall exposure to high levels of noise. Finally, hearing conservation programs, made up of regular audiometric testing of employees, hearing protection equipment policies, and workers' education, can go a long way toward creating a safer, quieter workplace.

References

1. National Institute for Occupational Safety and Health (NIOSH). 1991. *NIOSH Publications on Noise and Hearing.* Cincinnati: NIOSH.
2. National Institute for Occupational Safety and Health (NIOSH). 1988. *Proposed National Strategies for the Prevention of Leading Work-Related Diseases and Injuries: Noise-Induced Hearing Loss.* Cincinnati: NIOSH.
3. Ibid.
4. Starck, J. et al. 1995. "Factors Explaining Individual Variability in Hearing Levels: Exposure to Noise, Hearing Protection, Blood Pressure and Cholesterol." *Sixth US–Finnish Joint Symposium on Occupational Safety and Health.* Helsinki: Finnish Institute of Occupational Health.
5. Tubbs, Randy L. 1995. "Noise and Hearing Loss in Firefighting." *Occupational Medicine: State of the Art Reviews* 10:4 Philadelphia: Hanley & Belfus, Inc..
6. Lusk, Sally L., Madeleine J. Kerr and Sirkka A. Kauffman. 1998. "Use of Hearing Protection and Perceptions of Noise Exposure and Hearing Loss Among Construction Workers." *AIHA Journal* 59:7.

7. Ibid.
8. Early, Karen and S. W. Horstman. 1996. "Noise Exposure to Musicians During Practice." *Applied Occupational and Environmental Hygiene* 11:9.
9. Xing, J.J. et al. 1992. "Occupational Noise Exposure and Noise-Induced Hearing Loss: An Epidemiological Study in China Coal Miners." *Proceedings of the 9th. International Symposium on Epidemiology in Occupational Health*. Cincinnati: NIOSH.
10. Lawanson, S. and U. G. Oleru. 1992. "Temporary Hearing Threshold Levels in an Iron and Steel Factory in Nigeria." *Proceedings of the 9th. International Symposium on Epidemiology in Occupational Health*. Cincinnati: NIOSH.

CHAPTER 9

Skin Deep

Ann stood at the sink, rinsing off dishes. Through the window, she could see the lawn man unrolling the sprayer from his truck, but she didn't pay him much attention, her thoughts turning instead to her son. It had been Ryan who had found the lifeless form of the puppy lying in the grass yesterday. She didn't know why the pup had died.

Ryan was at a birthday party, but Ann knew that the party would make him happy for only a little while. He would still have to deal with his grief when he returned home.

Outside, the lawn man was walking back and forth across the lawn, spraying something he promised would kill the bugs that were destroying the grass.

She was placing the last of the dishes into the dishwasher when she heard what sounded like rain pattering against the wall. She looked outside and saw the lawn man waving the spray carelessly over the grass, at times running the spray up against the house. She noticed that he was unsteady and she wondered if maybe he was drunk or on drugs.

Just another thing to deal with she thought angrily, as she went out to talk to the man. When she was close enough to observe his face, he didn't appear to be drunk or high after all. She saw that he was pale and his eyes were unable to focus clearly. She didn't know what a sunstroke victim looked like but she thought maybe he was one.

"Are you all right?" she said. "Maybe you should sit down for a minute."

He smiled weakly. "Just the heat, I guess. I do feel a little woozy." He sat on the porch step. "Could I trouble you for a glass of water, maybe?"

She brought him the water and he sipped at it, resting in the shade of the porch. After a few minutes, he had recovered enough to go back to finishing the lawn treatment.

From inside the house she watched him work. He seemed to be all right, although he moved slowly. It took him some time to roll the hose back onto the truck, and when he backed the truck out of the driveway, he rolled over a corner of the lawn and almost hit the mailbox.

Ann saw the truck weave as it went down the street. Maybe he was on drugs after all, she thought. She didn't need that kind of man working around her house. She called the lawn care company on the phone and canceled her contract.

She didn't know that while she was on the phone, the lawn man sideswiped a car only a few miles from her home, almost causing a serious accident.

The skin is the largest organ of the human body, charged with keeping our innards where they belong and protecting them from infection or injury, and serving also as the body's thermostat. Because large surfaces of the skin are often directly exposed to the environment, this organ is particularly vulnerable to occupational diseases and injuries. Since trauma is discussed more completely in Chapter Eleven, this chapter will confine itself only to the broad category of skin disease, including diseases of the mucous membranes in the nose, mouth, and eyes.

There are several types of skin disorders caused by occupational factors; various skin cancers have been attributed to workplace conditions, although relatively few epidemiological studies exist. Contact dermatitis, a less serious disorder than cancer, is an inflammation of the skin caused either by some irritant agent or by some substance to which the worker is allergic. Various skin cancers have been attributed to workplace conditions, although relatively few epidemiological studies exist.

The skin also provides an important route of absorption for toxic chemical substances such as those found in pesticides, which result in systemic toxicity. Percutaneous absorption of a toxic pesticide is what made the lawn man sick and killed Ryan's puppy.

The Problem

The Bureau of Labor Statistics Annual Survey for 1984 showed that dermatological diseases accounted for 34 percent of all cases of chronic occupational disease, with the greatest number of cases occurring in the manufacturing industry.[1] An occupational cause for skin disease is easy to identify since there is visible evidence of the disorder. But it is often difficult to determine whether or not other diseases are a result of percutaneous absorption of toxins in the workplace; there are no reliable numbers available that can tell us how much of a problem percutaneous absorption may be. In a selected sample of hospital emergency room visits from 1981 to 1985, the National Electronic Injury Surveillance System found only three cases of acute systemic reactions that could be attributed to percutaneous absorption.[2] Still, this does not mean the problem does not exist, only that it is difficult to recognize since there are no visible signs on the skin and the symptoms may mimic other diseases.

Let's take a closer look at the various types of occupational skin diseases.

Contact dermatitis—Simply stated, contact dermatitis is an inflammation of the skin characterized by redness, itching, and various skin lesions caused by some physical agent. Irritant contact dermatitis is caused by physical contact with an irritating substance. Irritant contact dermatitis may be caused by apparently innocuous substances that we use in our daily lives such as soap, perfume, or deodorant. The familiar "dishpan hands" is a form of irritant contact dermatitis. The workplace, however, is filled with a greater and stronger variety of irritant agents.

Irritant contact dermatitis in the workplace may be caused by contact with soaps, detergents, miscellaneous cleaning products, solvents, food products, plastics and resins, and hard, particulate dusts (fibrous glass as an example). The resulting dermatitis commonly occurs on the hands, arms, and other skin surfaces that may come in contact with the substance, but the reaction does not usually spread to other parts of the body. It is frequently described as chafing, rash, or chapping. Although most cases of irritant contact dermatitis occur when the skin is in direct contact with the irritant, it can occur as a result of a secondary exposure. It is important to note that even contact with surfaces, objects, or clothes that are grossly contaminated by an irritant may result in this skin disorder. Sometimes, workplace irritants may have an additive effect. That is, contact with one or more different substances in the workplace could result in a chemical reaction that causes dermatitis.

While any worker with frequent, repeated contact to skin irritants can develop dermatitis, there are some individuals for whom the risk is greater. Persons with other skin conditions, such as psoriasis, or who have skin infections or injuries, are at greater risk of developing contact dermatitis. Workers with a personal or family history of atopy (allergies that are inherited, occurring in about 25 percent of the population) also have an increased risk, possibly 13-fold higher, compared to nonatopic individuals.

Allergic contact dermatitis is different from irritant contact dermatitis in that a worker must be sensitized to the irritant in order to develop a reaction. In nature, poison ivy and poison oak are irritants that will produce dermatitis in individuals who are sensitive to the plants. Many people develop reactions to poison ivy or poison oak, but the severity of their reaction will be determined by their degree of sensitivity to the plants. Some lucky people are not affected by these plants at all. In allergic dermatitis, one worker may have a reaction to something in the workplace while his coworkers do not. This is important to note because employers may think one individual's complaint is imagined or even faked.

The workplace holds many substances to which some people will develop an allergic contact dermatitis. Unlike irritant contact dermatitis, it may take only small amounts of the substance to produce a reaction among sensitized workers. It is also not uncommon to find the reaction on parts of the body that did not necessarily have contact with the substance. Indirect contact with objects, surfaces, and clothing that contain only a trace of the offending substance may still be sufficient enough to trigger widespread, severe dermatitis.

Some of the more common workplace substances that may produce allergic contact dermatitis among sensitized workers are: metallic salts, such as nickel, chromate, cobalt, gold, and mercury; plastics and resins; organic dyes, including photographic color developers; rubber accelerators and antioxidants; industrial biocides and germicides, such as formaldehyde and glutaraldehyde; and ironically, some first-aid preparations, including bacitracin, benzocaine, Mercurochrome, neomycin, and thimerosal.

The fact that contact dermatitis may be caused by either an irritant agent or by allergy means that it is difficult to determine a causative factor in a given workplace. Since allergies are so subjective, almost anyone may develop dermatitis, anyone from the butcher and baker to the candlestick maker.

Butcher—antibiotics, bacteria, brine, cold, detergents, enzymes, fungi, moisture, and parasites

Baker—benzoyl peroxide, cinnamon, dough, dusts, flavoring oils, flour, fungi, heat, moisture, spices, and sugar

Candlestick maker—ammonium salts, borax, boric acid, chlorine, chromates, hydrochloric acid, potassium nitrate, sodium hydroxide, stearic acid, and waxes

There are some industries and jobs that have an obvious potential for contact dermatitis. Workers in housekeeping, janitorial, and other cleaning services industries are at risk of developing contact dermatitis from soaps, detergents, and cleaning agents. Painters, mechanics, chemical workers, and machinists who use solvents in their daily tasks are also at risk. Food handlers and processors, as well as cooks, restaurant workers, and grocers, could develop contact dermatitis from some foods, as well as cleaning agents. Industrial and medical chemical laboratory workers using formaldehyde and other chemicals may be at risk of developing an allergic contact dermatitis. Denturists, their staff, and their patients have experienced contact dermatitis caused by methyl methacrylate monomer, a resin used in manufacturing dentures. Nurses and other hospital workers involved in disinfecting instruments with glutaraldehyde or similar agents may also develop an allergic dermatitis.

Another skin ailment common to health care workers is allergic dermatitis caused by exposure to latex, a milky fluid derived from the rubber tree, *Hevea brasiliensis*. Latex is widely used in surgical gloves and other medical products and also has many other nonmedical uses. In June 1997, the National Institute for Occupational Safety and Health (NIOSH) issued a public health alert that states, "Workers exposed to latex gloves and other products containing natural rubber latex may develop allergic reactions such as skin rashes; nasal, eye, or sinus symptoms; asthma; and (rarely) shock."[3] In addition to allergic reactions to latex, workers may also experience a simple contact dermatitis from the substance as well as an allergic contact dermatitis to some of the chemicals that are added to latex during harvesting, processing, or manufacturing.

It is estimated that up to 17 percent of health care workers are allergic to latex, and as much as 6 percent of the general population.[4] This latter percent will no doubt increase, as the AIDS threat has resulted in workers in other industries besides health care donning latex gloves to protect themselves from contracting the disease. Cosmetologists and hairdressers, police/fire/EMS personnel, food service workers, and housekeeping personnel are just some of the occupations at risk of latex-induced skin disorders.

It might seem that the solution to the latex problem is to ban latex in the workplace and in health care settings particularly. This is not as easy as it sounds. Latex is used in 40,000 products, including such common products as rubber bands, erasers, electric cords, and elastic in clothing. The product has its share of supporters in the health care industry, where it is widely used; surgeons and other medical professionals like the tactile sensitivity that latex gloves give them and latex is an effective barrier against blood-borne diseases. Vinyl and nitrile gloves are currently in use as latex substitutes, but it is not yet certain that these types of gloves will completely replace latex.

The latex problem is not a minor one. Workers at risk of developing latex allergies also tend to have multiple allergic reactions, including allergies to foods such as avocados, potatoes, bananas, papayas, and tomatoes. Some cases of latex dermatitis have been so severe as to end careers. Using nonirritating gloves and getting proper medical treatment are essential in protecting people from latex allergies.

Whether or not a worker develops a contact dermatitis as a result of an occupational irritant, or from an allergic reaction caused by a workplace substance, his prognosis is poor. Published reports suggest that only 25 percent of affected persons recover fully and completely while 50 percent improve but require intermittent treatment to maintain control, and the remaining 25 percent stay the same or worsen.[5]

Skin cancer—Since occupational cancers are discussed at length in Chapter Three, we will not spend too much time here on the subject. There have been relatively few epidemiological studies on the relationship of skin cancer to occupational exposures, but there is a great deal of evidence that establishes ultraviolet radiation as the most potent and important cutaneous carcinogen.

Although the current data is not precise, as much as 20 percent of the American workforce may be subjected to solar radiation for at least part of the day.[6] It makes sense, therefore, that persons who work outdoors in industries such as farming, construction, landscaping, gardening, nursery work, forestry, and road building may be at an increased risk of developing skin cancer.

Ultraviolet radiation may also be a problem on a job site, as in a welder's arc or in curing wood surface coatings. The health effects of ultraviolet radiation will vary, depending upon the wavelength and intensity of the exposure. In a study of workers involved in the process of curing coatings such as lacquers and paints on wood surfaces, ultraviolet radiation from the curing units was high enough to cause burns and keratitis within seconds.[7]

Personal susceptibility and differences in skin pigmentation play important roles in the development of skin cancer. Risks appear to be greater among fair-skinned individuals, who sunburn easily, compared to individuals with more heavily pigmented skin. Also, trauma to the skin, especially burns, may set the stage on rare occasions for skin cancer.

In addition to skin cancer caused by the effects of ultraviolet radiation, carcinogenic agents in the workplace that enter the body through percutaneous absorption, such as pesticides, may be linked to certain types of skin cancer.

Infections—There is a whole gardenful of microorganisms that can cause skin infections, including bacteria, fungi, viruses, and parasites. It is estimated that up to 5 percent of all workers' compensation claims for skin diseases are a result of skin infections. While some skin infections may be the result of injuries or the difficulty in keeping the skin clean on certain jobs, most of them are due to exposure to infectious microorganisms.

Specific occupations show an increased potential for exposure to these infectious critters. Fishermen, fish processors, and meat handlers may develop a skin infection, known as erysipeloid, caused by bacteria in fish and meat. Fishermen and aquarium workers may be infected by mycobacteria. Sheep and goat ranchers may develop orf, a pustular lesion on the finger, contracted from infected lambs, while wool handlers may contract anthrax from the hair, hides, or waste of sheep. Milker's nodule, similar to orf, is found in dairymen, and grain-mite itch is found in grain farmers. Gardeners and nursery workers may develop sporotrichosis, an infection characterized by abscesses, nodules, and ulcers, caused by the fungus *Sporotrichum schenckii*. Ringworm of the foot is often found in miners. Herpes simplex, an infectious disease that produces vesicles (little blisters) on the gums, in the throat, or the conjunctiva of the eye, poses a potential risk for dentists, nurses, physicians, and other health care workers. Epidemics of scabies, a highly communicable disease carried by the itch mite, is an occupational hazard for health workers, especially those working with patients with impaired immunity, AIDS, or with severe mental retardation.

Excessive heat and humidity, as well as constrictive clothing, may subject some workers to bacterial infections. The same may be said for cuts, burns, and abrasions.

Percutaneous absorption—Although it is not, itself, a skin disease, percutaneous absorption is the route through which some disease-causing toxins enter the body. These toxins may enter the body through direct skin contact with raw materials, contaminated work surfaces, or from toxins accidentally created in various manufacturing processes.

Percutaneous absorption is a common route for many insecticides to enter the body. Insecticide makers, farmers, gardeners, lawn care personnel, groundskeepers, and golf course workers are all at risk of disease, most notably cancer and central nervous system disorders, being delivered to them through percutaneous absorption.

A study sponsored by the Golf Course Superintendent Association showed significantly increased mortality rates caused by cancer; the group of superintendents in the study also showed a high number of deaths from diseases of the nervous system.[8] This same pattern of diseases has been shown in other workers occupationally exposed to pesticides. The most common route of entry for the toxic chemicals found in pesticides was through the skin of the hands and face while applying the pesticide through a sprayer.

Solvents, too, may enter the body through percutaneous absorption. A study of 97 auto body repair workers showed that dermal exposures to solvents contributed significantly to the total dosage of solvents absorbed by the workers.[9] The amount of xylene absorbed by the body through hand contact with the solvent, even in as short a time period as 15 minutes, was greater than the amount of xylene the workers received from inhalation over a full shift.

Percutaneous absorption of toxic chemicals may be enhanced in workers with skin trauma (cuts, abrasions, burns) or who have had prolonged skin contact with the chemical. Workers with existing dermatitis or wet or hot skin, such as the lawn man, may also be at an increased risk of chemical toxicity through percutaneous absorption. Some common toxic chemicals that may be absorbed through the skin are aniline, benzene, cyanide salts, and mercury, a substance that because of its quirky physical properties was sometimes used as a plaything.

While it stretches the definition of percutaneous absorption somewhat, this is a good time to talk about diseases among health care workers that are the result of accidental needle sticks. When contaminated needles are lost, left lying around, or disposed of improperly the possibility exists for a health care worker to accidentally stick himself with the needle and thus expose himself to the possibility of contracting an infectious disease. There are already several documented cases in which health care workers have contracted the AIDS virus through such accidents.

Hepatitis may also be spread through accidental sticks with contaminated needles and in fact is a greater threat than AIDS. Far more health care workers die each year from hepatitis contracted through accidental needle sticks than they do from AIDS contracted in the same manner. These hepatitis deaths had been occurring for years; only now, because of the high-profile AIDS threat, is the hepatitis issue being addressed. There are protocols established for the safe disposal of used needles, and we cannot overstate the importance of adhering to them.

Miscellaneous skin diseases—There are several skin diseases and disorders that may be caused by workplace conditions that do not fit neatly into any of the above categories. Some of the more common ones are:

- **Acne**—includes tropical acne from heat and moisture, a major cause of early military discharges from Vietnam; occupational acne, sometimes called "McDonald's acne," caused by oils and grease; and chloracne from dioxin and related chemicals
- **Leukoderma**—a depigmentation of the skin resulting in white patches; hydroquinone, used in shopping mall rapid development of black-and-white film, is one culprit
- **Hyperpigmentation**—caused by repeated trauma and rubbing of the skin and commonly seen in produce workers
- **Nail diseases**—includes chronic paronychia (infection around the nail) caused by repeated immersion of the fingertips in water, especially hot water, seen in bartenders, kitchen workers, and laundry workers; onycholysis (detachment of the nail from its bed) experienced by laundry workers and hairdressers;

koilonychia (a condition in which the fingernail becomes concave; "spoon nail") caused by solvents and oils that weaken the nails and make them more susceptible to malformation; Bowen's disease (squamous cell carcinoma)

- **Urticaria**—symptoms range from itching, swelling, and edema to anaphylaxis and even death; it may be allergic as in latex allergies or may be telangiectasia, a disorder caused by chronic exposure to sunlight
- **Photosensitivity**—may be a phototoxic reaction in which a chemical in the body reacts to sunlight—some phototoxic reactions may last for months or even years; some who may experience these reactions are workers who harvest celery, grocery workers and chefs who handle celery, and roofers and pitch workers; photoallergic reactions have been noted in nurses, hospital laundry workers, and pharmacists who administer phenothiazines or are exposed to these active drugs in patients' body secretions, notably urine
- **Miliaria**—obstruction of the sweat glands and sweat retention caused by high humidity in the workplace.

Workplace demographics in the U.S. are changing and current risk patterns may be altered by these changes. As we near the year 2000, current trends indicate declining worker populations in agriculture and a shift from heavy to light manufacturing, both of which may lower the number of workers exposed to conditions that cause skin disease. Still, new technologies and new occupations may mean new forms of skin disease for a segment of the population not currently affected.

Mucous membranes—The mucous membranes of the nose, mouth, and eyes also present an additional pathway for workplace diseases to enter the body. Frequently, these membranes are irritated by exposures to various irritants and the worker will complain of an odd taste in his mouth, or perhaps stinging eyes or nasal irritation. These complaints may seem minor, but they need to be recognized as indicators of exposure to a potentially harmful chemical. Sometimes, disease of the mucous membranes can lead to a serious medical condition and even death.

In October 1997, a 22-year-old female laboratory technician working at the Yerkes Regional Primate Research Center in Lawrenceville, Georgia, contracted a case of *Herpesvirus simiae*, or "B" virus, and died two months later.[10] The Occupational Safety and Health Administration (OSHA) investigated the death and found that the technician was conducting experiments with macaque monkeys, primates who are known to harbor the "B" virus in their blood, bodily secretions, and tissues. While transferring one of the monkeys from a transfer box into a cage, she was splashed in the eye with urine and diarrhea from the animal. She immediately wiped her eye with a paper towel and flushed it with water 45 minutes later; she did not file an incident report. Her death on December 10 was a direct result of the "B" virus contracted in her workplace.

The tragic part of this bizarre fatality is that it could have easily been avoided by the use of the proper protective clothing. One of the several citations OSHA lodged against Yerkes was for the laboratory's failure to provide either protective goggles or face shields for its technicians, a simple precaution that would have saved the young woman's life.

Developing a Thick Hide

A person who is not easily aggravated by criticism or insults is said to have a "thick hide." In order for you to reduce your risk of contracting a skin disease in the workplace, you, too, need to develop a thick hide.

Obviously, the best way to protect yourself from skin disease is to make sure that every possible cause of disease is eliminated in your workplace. This means isolating some equipment and machinery that may cause disease, and eliminating toxic chemicals entirely, or substituting them with nontoxic chemicals. The same can be accomplished for contact allergens.

While these changes are obvious, in all probability you may not have the authority, and perhaps the knowledge, to carry them out. They are changes that need to come from top management, and that may be a difficult process. As is so often the case, some of the changes necessary to create a safer workplace may be costly and might cut into profits. Top management, always answering to the stockholders first, may find that spending money for a safer workplace is not a sound business decision, especially when the company may be in compliance with OSHA standards. And, to be fair to the company, there may be certain processes or chemicals necessary to the industry that simply cannot be substituted for safer methods, or for which no safer alternatives exist. There may not be much you can do about engineering controls in your workplace to reduce the incidence of skin disease other than working through supervisors or union representatives to try and make changes, but there are steps you can take to reduce your personal vulnerability to skin disease.

Personal protective equipment, especially gloves and splash guards such as goggles and face shields, is justified only when a health hazard cannot be corrected either through substitution or engineering and administrative controls, as mentioned above. If your job requires protective equipment, you should ask yourself, and your employer as well, if all other corrective options have been exhausted. Is protective equipment the only way you can be safeguarded against dangerous exposures?

If protective equipment proves necessary, it is very important to make sure that the proper equipment is selected. Analyze the specific task for which the equipment is to be used and understand exactly what it should do to protect you. For example, if gloves are needed, what type of gloves should they be? Latex? Vinyl? Nitrile? These types of gloves have varying degrees of permeability, strength, and tactile sensation, and so should be chosen based upon the task to be performed. It is equally important to make sure the equipment is right for you specifically. Do the gloves fit properly? Are you allergic to their material?

It may seem unnecessary—how many different ways can you put on a glove?—but a training program for the proper use of protective equipment should be established. As an example, making sure your hands are clean before putting on your gloves can help to reduce your risk of contracting a skin disorder. The program should detail exactly when to use protective equipment, for how long, and should cover care and maintenance of the equipment. Proper maintenance is as important as the proper selection; equipment that is dirty, contaminated, or damaged may fail to protect you adequately.

If protective equipment is required in your workplace, then there must be an enforcement policy in place to make sure that everyone is following the rules. We all know by now to buckle our seat belts in an airplane, yet the flight attendant still calls it to our attention on every flight and the plane will not take off until everyone is buckled in; that same type of reminder needs to take place in the workplace when it comes to wearing protective equipment.

Finally, there needs to be an ongoing evaluation of the protective equipment and how it is used by the workers. Supervisors should make spot checks and not simply hand out the equipment and assume it is used. Personal protective equipment programs may need to be fine-tuned to make sure the protective equipment is effective.

Wearing the proper protective clothing recommended for your particular workplace is essential. Whether the clothing is as simple as gloves and safety glasses or as complex as full-body suits, if it is recommended for your job, you should wear it. Vanity and looking "cool" have no place on the job. Your health is your number one priority.

Although the study pertained to injury, rather than disease, the Bureau of Labor Statistics found that only 1 percent of workers suffering facial injuries and 17 percent of workers sustaining head injuries were wearing the appropriate protective clothing at the time. Similar patterns may be shown for workers wearing chemical protective clothing.

Chemical protective clothing itself may cause or aggravate dermatitis. Sweat trapped in the clothing and skin rubbing against it could cause irritation, as could chemicals accidentally trapped in the clothing. Sometimes, contact allergies may result from the clothing. A common example of this is an allergic reaction caused by chemical additives in latex gloves. Still, chemical protective clothing should be worn wherever appropriate.

In addition to protective clothing, there has been a great deal of research on barrier creams, substances that can be applied to the skin in order to block out harmful chemicals or irritants. Sunscreens with high solar protection factors (SPF) are examples of barrier creams that have been shown to be extremely effective, against ultraviolet radiation in this case. The verdict is still out, though, on the use of barrier creams in the manufacturing industry. What benefits seem to arise from the use of these creams are anecdotal and may result from the lubricating effect on the skin that the creams provide, or from improved personal hygiene, or a reduced need for skin washing, rather than from any chemical action. This is not to imply that effective barrier creams may not be developed, only that the data currently indicates they have not yet been perfected.

Good personal hygiene is an effective way to help reduce your risk of skin disease in the workplace. Washing with water alone is generally enough for skin contact with acids and alkalies. Specific decontamination procedures exist for certain chemicals in order to prevent chemical burns, and you should be knowledgeable about them if you are working with any of these chemicals. Some common examples of these chemicals are hydrofluoric acid, phenol, alkyl mercury compounds, white phosphorus, and chromic acid.

References

1. National Institute for Occupational Safety and Health (NIOSH). 1988. *Proposed Strategies for the Prevention of Leading Work-Related Diseases and Injuries.* Cincinnati: NIOSH.
2. Ibid.
3. National Institute for Occupational Safety and Health (NIOSH). 1997. *Preventing Allergic Reactions to Natural Rubber Latex in the Workplace.* Cincinnati: NIOSH.
4. Kedjidjian, Catherine B. "Get the Facts About Latex." *Safety + Health* May 1998.
5. National Institute for Occupational Safety and Health (NIOSH). 1988. *Proposed Strategies for the Prevention of Leading Work-Related Diseases and Injuries.* Cincinnati: NIOSH.
6. Ibid.

7. Surakka, Jouni et al. 1997. "Assessment of Ultraviolet Radiation Exposure in the Wood Surface Coating Industry." *Applied Occupational and Environmental Hygiene* 12:4.
8. Kross, Burton C., Howard F. Nicholson and Linda K. Ogilvie. 1996. "Methods Development Study for Measuring Pesticide Exposure to Golf Course Workers Using Video Imaging Techniques." *Applied Occupational and Environmental Hygiene* 11:11.
9. Daniell, William et al. 1992. "The Contribution to Solvent Uptake by Skin and Inhalation Exposure." *American Industrial Hygiene Association Journal* 53:2.
10. Occupational Safety and Health Administration (OSHA). Internet *News Release* April 27, 1998.

CHAPTER 10

Your Aching Back

It wasn't the most interesting summer job Dennis had ever worked, but the hours were good. He had his evenings free so he could still visit the dance clubs in town with his friends. Dennis loved to dance. In fact, he always had to be in motion. If he wasn't on the dance floor, he'd be shooting hoops, or jogging in the park, anything to keep his body moving. Dennis was energetic, always in a rush, his friends said, and sometimes he was in too much of a hurry to think before he acted.

His job in the receiving section at the department store kept him busy most of the time. He loaded and unloaded trucks, brought boxes of merchandise to the various departments in the store, packed goods for transfer to other stores, and did whatever else was asked of him.

Dennis noticed that some of the older guys on the loading dock wore back-support belts and he was vaguely aware of the wall chart that showed the proper way to lift a heavy load, but somehow those precautions didn't seem directed toward him. He was 20 years old and in great shape; it was the old geezers who had to be careful.

A truck from an electronics distributor was in the dock and several televisions and boxes of stereo equipment had already been off-loaded onto a cart for delivery to the floor. Dennis grabbed the handle of the cart and pushed it from the dock to the freight elevator. At the second floor, he wheeled the cart over to the electronics department and began to remove the smaller boxes of stereo equipment from the cart. Once they were stacked on the floor, he reached for one of the televisions.

The box wasn't that large, but one side felt heavier than the other, a fact he didn't notice until he had already taken hold of the box and yanked it up off the cart. Instantly, he felt a pain in his lower back so sharp that it felt as though someone had stabbed him from behind. The box slipped from his fingers and fell back on the cart.

He stood by the cart, bent slightly forward, trying to regain his breath. His back seemed locked into an iron straitjacket that had been made red-hot in the fires of hell.

"Hey, man, are you okay?"

From the corner of his eye, Dennis saw Matt, one of the loading-dock crew.

"No," he said, between clenched teeth, "I can't move."

Matt was afraid to move his friend, so he had store security call for the paramedics. Two hours later, Dennis was beginning to feel better, a result of the muscle relaxants he had been given in the hospital emergency room.

As he lay on the gurney, Dennis wondered how soon it would be before he was dancing again.

Back injuries similar to Dennis's are not uncommon in the workplace. A 1977 survey conducted by the National Center for Health Statistics estimated that 19 million persons suffered musculoskeletal injuries on the job.[1] While the survey showed greater risks for injury in manufacturing, construction, and food processing industries, it also found that nearly one-half of all U.S. workers are affected by musculoskeletal injuries sometime during their working life.

The survey further indicated that musculoskeletal injuries, because of their ability to limit physical activity, rank first among health problems in the frequency in which they affect the quality of life.

"Musculoskeletal disorders are among the most prevalent medical problems in the U.S., affecting 7 percent of the population. They account for 14 percent of physician visits and 19 percent of hospital stays," said Dr. Linda Rosenstock, National Institute for Occupational Safety and Health (NIOSH) Director.[2]

The cost of these injuries as measured in lost earnings and workers' compensation is enormous. The Bureau of Labor Statistics estimates that the cost of cumulative trauma disorders alone may be as high as $100 billion.[3] At least one-third of all workers' compensation claims annually are for musculoskeletal injuries, with sprains and strains the most prevalent. Back injuries account for about 50 percent of these complaints, followed by injuries to the ankle, knee, and shoulder.

The high incidence of musculoskeletal injuries in the workplace has spawned the new science of ergonomics, which studies how a job can be fit to human anatomical, physiological, and psychological characteristics in order to enhance human efficiency and well-being.

The Problem

Let's define what we mean by musculoskeletal injuries. NIOSH considers these disorders to be both acute and chronic injuries to muscles, tendons, ligaments, nerves, joints, bones, and the supporting vasculature; injuries such as sprains, strains, inflammations, irritations, and dislocations. NIOSH defines injuries in which the skin or bones are broken as a result of the transfer of high energy—as from a fall—as traumatic injuries, which will be discussed in Chapter Eleven.

In order for a particular musculoskeletal injury to be considered work-related, there must be some type of biomechanical stress, a traumatogen, involved. Repetitive or sustained lifting, heavy lifting, bending, twisting, climbing, reaching, gripping, pinching, rubbing, kneeling, and squatting, as well as equipment vibrations, are all common traumatogens. Frequently, these activities are performed in awkward positions and involve heavy force, thereby increasing the risk of injury.

Since musculoskeletal injuries can affect any of us, at any time, whether at work or not, it is not always easy to pinpoint a workplace traumatogen as the sole cause of such an injury. Sole cause or not, the workplace remains an environment with great potential for injury. Our lives complicate injury in the workplace and vice versa. Many a sore "weekend warrior" has gone into work on Monday and suffered a muscle strain leading to injury that normally would not have bothered him. Other personal conditions, such as anatomy, physical fitness, previous injuries, and age-related changes, make us even more vulnerable to musculoskeletal injuries in the workplace.

More specifically, certain human biological factors can affect a worker's vulnerability to such injuries. Physical size, strength, flexibility, and stamina are all important factors and when the worker's capacity in these areas does not match the demands of the job, injury may result.

Behavioral and lifestyle factors can also determine a worker's vulnerability to injury. Too little sleep and too much exertion can affect job performance adversely and put the worker in harm's way. Psychological factors such as perceiving the job as too demanding or too hazardous, or simply being dissatisfied with the job, can have the same effect. Mental lapses, brought on by workplace exposures to stress and chemicals, or through the use of drugs and alcohol, can impair a worker's judgment on the job, sometimes with severe consequences. Obesity and poor physical fitness are obvious risks in suffering a musculoskeletal injury.

Another important factor that contributes to injury is the worker's lack of knowledge either about workplace hazards or about preventive methods of avoiding injury. Sometimes, it is not lack of knowledge, but a stubborn refusal to obey safe working practices that may cause this type of injury.

Musculoskeletal injuries in the workplace can be broadly classified in two groups, those that affect the back, especially the lower back, and those that affect the extremities. Lower back pain is a common enough ailment on the job, but it is often difficult to determine what causes it, or to isolate a single workplace factor as being responsible. As in other occupational disorders, the overall health and lifestyle of the individual worker must be taken into consideration in order to find out specifically what role workplace factors play in his injury. This is especially true with lower back pain, as ubiquitous an injury as can be found on the job.

But is that lower back pain the result of tossing packages into the back of a delivery truck all day or is it the result of pulling weeds from the garden over the weekend? Or is it some combination of both? Current theory holds that there are some identifiable workplace factors that can indeed contribute to lower back pain. These include load weight, location of the load, how often materials are handled, and vibration from equipment used on the job (studies have shown a relationship between lower back pain and seat vibrations among operators of agricultural tractors, freight-container tractors, forklift trucks, and helicopters).[4]

Other factors that contribute to lower back injuries are fatigue, stress (both physical and emotional), trauma, degenerative changes, congenital defects, neurological dysfunction, and genetics.

While workplace factors for lower back injuries are fairly well documented, the same cannot be said for injuries to the extremities. Some progress has been made, however, in determining workplace causes of injury to the upper extremities. Studies of hand and arm motions on the job have been helpful in identifying points of stress, especially relative to carpal tunnel syndrome and tenosynovitis (inflammation of the sheath surrounding a tendon).

Studies of the lower extremities, however, have been limited almost exclusively to the knee. Workplace factors that have been connected to knee injury include constant kneeling or squatting, and repetitive loading, as well as repetitive contact between the knee and tools used on the job.

There are certain industries in which one would expect to find a high rate of musculoskeletal injuries. Construction, manufacturing, farming, and logging are just a few. One industry that has been studied at some length, relative to the rate of workplace injuries, is the meatpacking industry.

Upton Sinclair's book, *The Jungle*, published in 1906, was an exposé of the meatpacking industry, vividly describing its squalor, unsanitary environment, and thoroughly unsafe working conditions. Sinclair's graphic depictions of Chicago slaughterhouses so revolted the public (President Teddy Roosevelt is said to have thrown his breakfast sausages out a window after reading the book) that the U.S.

Congress passed the Pure Food and Drug Act that same year, as well as the Meat Inspection Act.

In addition to the workplace environment itself, Sinclair wrote about the workers, who went about their jobs in a mad rush, laboring with little regard for their own health or safety. Brandishing razor-sharp knives, they concentrated only on keeping the disassembly line moving at all costs.

Meatpackers today still work at a frenzied pace, sometimes making one cut every three seconds as they hack up animal carcasses. In such a hectic environment mistakes are made and workers are injured. In 1988, the Occupational Safety and Health Administration (OSHA) proposed a fine of $4.6 million against meatpacker John Morrell & Company for what the agency termed "egregious" and "willful" health violations at Morrell's plant in Sioux Falls, South Dakota.[5] Two years later, the company reached a settlement with OSHA for $990,000 in proposed penalties and further agreed to make a grant to NIOSH in the amount of $260,000 for continuing study of musculoskeletal injuries.

In another case the previous year, the U.S. Labor Department had fined Iowa Beef Packers $2.59 million for "willfully" failing to report 1,038 instances of workplace injuries and illnesses.[6]

Loading-dock workers are another group among whom musculoskeletal injuries are common, mostly caused by lifting excessive loads. In the 1980s, studies conducted by the Industrial Commission of Ohio found that the motor freight transportation and warehousing industries accounted for more back injuries than any other industry in the state.[7] Similarly, researchers in California found that more than half the injuries in the trucking industry were associated with loading and unloading trucks. A NIOSH study of workers in the shipping department at a cabinet manufacturing company revealed that 79 percent of the workers reported musculoskeletal pain or discomfort in the year previous to the study.[8]

The NIOSH study found that musculoskeletal injuries could be reduced through engineering controls such as the implementation of an automated palletization and truck loading system, the use of assisted-lifting devices, and by reducing the weight of individual boxes. Recommended administrative controls to reduce injuries included two-man lifting of heavier loads, more frequent rotation of workers from lifting tasks to lighter assignments, and limiting the need for staging of boxes before loading onto trucks, thereby reducing the number of times a box is lifted.

The risk of musculoskeletal disorders in the construction and building trades is a serious and costly one. The U.S. Bureau of Labor estimates that there are 226,000 injuries each year, resulting in lost time and requiring either restricted work duties or complete time off from the job.[9] Depending upon the trade, workers' compensation insurance premiums in the construction industry have ranged from 7 percent to well over 100 percent of payroll. In terms of workers' compensation, bricklayers, carpenters, and ironworkers have had the fastest-growing insurance costs over the last several years, with workers' compensation insurance costs for bricklayers averaging 19 percent of payroll. This increased cost of doing business, as in other industries, is then passed on to the consumer.

Typical musculoskeletal disorders among bricklayers primarily affect the back, neck, and shoulders, and secondarily the elbow, wrist, and hand. Carpenters suffer from musculoskeletal disorders caused by the three commonly cited ergonomic job risk factors: use of stressful postures, excessive forces, and highly repetitive motions.

While we might expect musculoskeletal injuries to occur in the above occupations, these types of injuries are occurring with greater regularity in workplaces that at first glance do not seem dangerous. As new technologies emerge in the workplace so do new types of injuries—arpal tunnel syndrome, for example.

Carpal tunnel syndrome is an injury that has been reported on the rise since the mid-1980s, concomitant with the increasing use of computers, video display terminals, optical scanners, and similar equipment in the workplace. It is one of the fastest-growing occupational illnesses in the United States, affecting workers in the meatpacking, newspaper, poultry, textile, and electronics industries, as well as thousands of office workers and computer operators.

Carpal tunnel syndrome is an example of a repetitive motion injury, an injury caused by repeated stress to an area of the body as a direct result of some work activity. In carpal tunnel syndrome, the median nerve in the hand is compressed at the point at which it passes through the carpal tunnel (the bones of the wrist), resulting in pain, numbness, or tingling in the hand along the median nerve. It is a very painful condition that may require surgery for correction. Generally, it is repetitiveness and wrist flexion or hyperextension that causes carpal tunnel syndrome, but other work-related factors such as high hand forces, vibration, stress exerted on the creases of the wrist, and cold temperatures also have an effect on the incidence of the syndrome.

Carpal tunnel syndrome is becoming prevalent among secretaries, computer programmers, service representatives—anyone who uses a computer—whose wrists are in a constant state of flexion and extension as they work the keyboard.

A study conducted by the Department of Epidemiology at the UCLA School of Public Health, University of California, Los Angeles, examined the incidence of carpal tunnel syndrome among workers from three California labor unions.[10] The 652 subjects in the first union were employed as office workers, data entry operators, court clerks, and office clerks. The second group was made up of 389 construction carpenters, and the third, 452 union sprinkler fitters. A self-administered questionnaire was mailed to the test subjects in which they were asked about the type and severity of symptoms (pain, tingling, and numbness in the wrist, hand, and/or fingers) they experienced on the job. The study showed that the prevalence of symptoms was highest among office workers (21.3 percent), followed by sprinkler fitters and carpenters.

As more and more people are working at home (most of them on computers) it is probable that carpal tunnel syndrome and other ergonomic disorders will become prevalent in home offices. Home office–based workers most likely will not invest in ergonomically designed office furniture and equipment because of the expense, and it is certain that these workers will not receive any ergonomic training other than what they manage to haphazardly pick up on their own. These workers may be at real risk of serious ergonomic problems.

As research continues and new technologies develop, more ergonomic disorders will be discovered. Conveyor belt vertigo is an example. In this poorly documented disorder, workers whose jobs require visual fixation on moving objects (inspectors, food packers, assembly line workers) sometimes feel a spinning sensation known as circular vection illusion. Meclizine or other antivertigo agents can be given to the worker, but one must wonder if those drugs will have an effect on his job performance.

The future looks bright for anyone planning a career in ergonomics.

Standing Tall

As in all occupational diseases, prevention requires examining both the work environment and the individual worker. In the case of musculoskeletal injuries, the workplace and the job requirements can frequently be connected directly to the incidence of injury. A big step toward worker safety and health, therefore, is for companies to alter the work environment in such a way that it becomes less of a risk to workers. There are several actions a company can take to establish a sound ergonomics program for its workers:

- A corporate ergonomics program must fully engage the workers since it is the employee himself who has to carry much of the responsibility for lowering the ergonomic risks associated with his job. After all, who would know better how that worker lifts a load or operates the equipment in his workplace? Who else would know if his work on a computer causes wrist pain or if his office chair causes back strain? Workers must be fully involved in any corporate ergonomics program in order for it to be successful. They must be taught the concepts of ergonomics and the importance of good ergonomic practices to their overall health.
- The company must accurately identify hazards in the workplace that may result in musculoskeletal injuries. Is there machinery that produces excessive vibration or that has continual contact with vulnerable parts of the body, such as the wrist, knee, and back? Are there machines or job tasks that require a significant amount of strength to operate or perform? What about machines or tasks that do not require brute strength but that do exert continual stress on bones, joints, and tendons? These machines do not produce an immediate, visible injury, and so may be considered safe,

when in fact continuous, unnoticed injuries are occurring. Eventually, their cumulative effects will be felt.

In workplaces where such machines and job tasks are found, the company needs to find ways to eliminate or reduce injuries associated with them. One way is to replace injury-causing machinery with newer, ergonomically designed machinery. This may not always be practical, however. Ergonomics is such a new science that its practical applications are only in their infancy. It is entirely possible that there may not yet be an ergonomically designed replacement available. If such machinery does exist, it could be expensive, in which case the company is put in the position of weighing the price of worker safety and health against profitability, a debate that doesn't always favor the worker. Still, many industries have found the cost of ergonomic solutions to be well worth the price, as they realize decreased medical costs, a reduction in lost time due to injuries, and greater productivity.

- The company needs to make sure that adequate worker training programs are in place and that they are *implemented.* It is one thing for a company to have a training program available but quite another for it to be used properly and consistently. When we speak of worker training, we are talking about the "how to" aspects of the job: how to safely operate a forklift or stack pallets, say, or how to handle hazardous chemicals. The educational component of the program gives the worker the "why" and attempts to teach him the health benefits that he can derive from carrying out his tasks in the proper way. Remember, no worker intentionally seeks to hurt himself and a better trained, better educated workforce is less likely to suffer injury.

There are a few questions company trainers need to ask themselves about their training and education program. Is every new hire being given proper training as soon as he is hired? Are veteran employees periodically checked to see if they are still complying with proper safety procedures? If a worker is reassigned to a new task, is he instructed on safety procedures for that job? Who does the training? A professional? Another worker?

A thorough safety training program will include information on how to recognize workplace hazards and will provide opportunities for workers to participate in problem-solving sessions that will help them control hazardous activities. This is very important; including workers in the problem-solving process helps the company arrive at solutions that are more likely to work since they have been arrived at, in part, by the people who actually experience the problems. Workers will be more apt to put these solutions into practice since they helped develop them, and they will perceive the company as being truly interested in their safety and well-being.

A good ergonomics training program will include the basics—lessons as simple as how a worker can adjust his chair for proper posture or arrange his computer and workstation to avoid strain—and will not take anything for granted when it comes to assessing the worker's knowledge of ergonomics.

While many companies establish and maintain their own safety training programs, NIOSH also has available a variety of training programs through its Educational Resource Centers. OSHA, as well, has some limited assistance available through their consultation services.

- When corrective actions (newly designed tools and equipment, changes in work practices, automation, etc.) are taken in the workplace to reduce ergonomic injuries, it is important that the company evaluate the efficacy of these measures through worker feedback. They should do this several times at intervals, in order to reduce what is known as the Hawthorne effect (a sort of placebo effect immediately after corrective measures are taken), so that the efficacy of the measures can be accurately determined.

- The company should make sure that the right worker is matched up with the right job. Should an 87-year-old grandmother be carrying bricks at a construction site? Probably not (at least not without a hard hat), and yet workers are often mismatched with their jobs, either because of age, gender, physical fitness, lifestyle, or overall health. In today's politically correct and antidiscriminatory environment, it may seem wrong to screen workers for certain jobs, but such screening offers a potential method of protecting a worker from injury. Sometimes, workers with identified risk factors may be given additional ergonomics training. In a similar vein, if workers on the job eventually realize that the physical demands of their tasks are beyond their capabilities, switching to another, less demanding job could help.
- The company should set up a program of aggressive medical management. It may be that in the early stages of musculoskeletal injuries the worker is first treated or examined by the company nurse or physician. Eventually, the worker will probably receive medical care from a practitioner not connected to the workplace. Unless that practitioner has a detailed understanding of his patient's work activities, he may not be able to properly diagnose the condition nor prescribe an appropriate course of treatment. It is important that the company maintain a dialogue with the worker while he is being treated to make sure that all the conditions of his injury are told to the practitioner.

- The company should look beyond the physical parameters of the workplace and examine its own psychological parameters, its corporate philosophies about work and productivity. Some companies may endorse the bodybuilder's false maxim, "no pain, no gain," as they exert pressure on their supervisors, and ultimately their workers, in an attempt to boost production levels. This "push" philosophy, trickling down from top management, looks for 101 percent productivity, and has little tolerance for achievements below that level. In such a workplace, mistakes will be made, workers will attempt to exceed their physical—to say nothing of mental—capabilities, and injuries will invariably occur.

  Is the answer in this case for companies to settle for a lower level of productivity? Does the end result of improved worker safety necessarily mean that the company may lose its competitive edge and see an erosion in its profitability? The answer to both questions is no. Working smarter may be more beneficial to both the company and its workers than working harder. The latter approach, with its resulting higher incidence of injuries, will create more downtime on the job caused by the loss of injured workers and will mean more workers' compensation claims. Working smarter by following successful safety procedures means more workers on the job at any given time and less of the company's profits lost through workers' compensation. In the long run, working smarter is a safe and cost-effective alternative to the "push" philosophy.

While we are advocating that corporate America take the initiative in developing ergonomic programs to protect its workforce, most corporations have no legal requirement to do so since there is no federal OSHA ergonomics standard in place (some state OSHAs, most notably California's CAL/OSHA, have standards in place for businesses in their states). OSHA has been working to develop an ergonomics standard but has been stalled by the ongoing debate among state and federal agencies and politicians about what the standard should include. It is impossible for OSHA to develop a standard that would address every conceivable ergonomic injury for every worker in every occupation. Most likely OSHA's standard will be programmatic and will probably include a focus on identifying and trying to eliminate ergonomic risks; worker ergonomic training and education; monitoring the effectiveness of corrective measures; and consulting with corporations' worker safety and health representatives to help formulate corrective measures.

Some industries and their political supporters are fighting both federal and state OSHAs' attempts to develop ergonomics standards on the basis that there is not yet enough scientific evidence proving the severity and prevalence of ergonomic disorders and that corrective measures would prove too costly to implement and would, therefore, jeopardize business. Texas representative Henry Bonilla is one legislator who has been blocking OSHA's attempts to develop an ergonomics standard; some restrictions organized by him include barring the agency from developing a rule and even from collecting data about ergonomic injuries.[11]

In California, the American Trucking Association and the California Trucking Association have been fighting the CAL/OSHA Standard Board's third version of an ergonomics proposal that would affect businesses with ten or more employees.[12]

However, OSHA is not completely toothless without an ergonomic standard. Under the agency's "general duty clause," OSHA can insist on corrective measures but it must first be able to prove that a serious hazard exists in the workplace, that the hazard is recognized as serious in that industry, and that there is a feasible way to correct it. These criteria are not always easily proven and corporations are often successful in challenging them in court.

On Your Own Two Feet

While the laws are still being developed, what can you do to reduce the risk of suffering a musculoskeletal injury at work? First, as has been stressed in every chapter of this book, know your workplace; we cannot overstate the importance of being an informed worker. Learn what stresses, what hazards exist for you at your job, and learn how to eliminate, avoid, or minimize them. Evaluate your workplace and the equipment or machinery you use to determine the risks of musculoskeletal injuries. Any place where your body comes into contact with these objects is a point of risk. Concrete floors offer a good example. Many workplaces, especially in the manufacturing industries, are equipped with bare concrete floors. Besides obvious injuries from falls on their hard surfaces, concrete floors can cause stress and strain on muscles and bones in the feet, legs, and back. You can reduce fatigue and heel strike simply by using a cushioned floormat or at least heel cups or cushioned insoles in your shoes; changing footwear during the course of the day may also help to reduce injury.

Part of knowing your workplace is knowing how to work smarter. Try to plan your daily tasks in such a way as to reduce physical effort. There is an old saying among safety officers that says "Never lift that which must be lowered." Keeping this saying in mind, try to keep your tasks, or your tools and materials, at the same elevation so as to reduce the potential for injury. If you must lift heavy objects, always try to use mechanical lifting devices whenever possible.

Second, use whatever safety devices are recommended for your job; back belts, wrist pads at keyboards, and knee pads are just a few. Safety devices should be available for your use if you work at a job with the potential for musculoskeletal injury, and if they are not, you should ask that such devices be brought into the workplace.

A quick update on the efficacy of back belts is necessary here. In a study of 36,000 employees of a national hardware chain who were mandated by company policy to wear back belts, a researcher from the UCLA School of Public Health in Los Angeles found a 34 percent drop in the incidence of lower back injuries but was not able to conclusively link that decrease to the use of back belts.[13]

Some researchers are concerned about increased injuries to the hips of back-belt wearers since the belts immobilize the lower back but create more force upon the hips; the energy expended in a particular manual task remains constant, no matter where it has its effect upon the body—if it does not affect the lower back, the energy will be transferred somewhere else. Other researchers think that the use of back belts may have more of a psychological effect than an actual one. It could be that a worker wearing a back belt is simply more aware of ergonomic problems and works in a more safe manner. In short, the jury is still out on the efficacy of back belts.

Third, it is important that you participate in safety training programs and that you put into practice what you have learned. Conscientiously thinking about your own personal safety on the job, while utilizing your knowledge and the appropriate safety devices, can help you avoid injury.

Fourth, you should fill out any incident report as clearly and completely as possible. Most companies ask workers to fill out an incident report when they sustain a workplace injury. These reports are reviewed by the company's safety officer and provide a valuable tool to understanding safety hazards in that workplace and how to remedy them. But the safety officer can only make judgments based upon the information the worker provides him. If the information is inaccurate or incomplete, erroneous judgments could be made about the safety of the workplace.

As an example, if a worker on a loading dock reports that he strained his back lifting a heavy box, the safety officer may conclude that the injury was the employee's fault: he tried to lift a weight beyond his capabilities or he did not observe proper lifting procedures, or maybe he was just out of shape. If, on the other hand, the worker reports that he was tired from working overtime hours and the boxes were piling up on the loading dock, both conditions a result of "push" philosophy as the company cranked up production levels, it becomes apparent to the safety officer that the worker is not necessarily at fault. The safety officer has found a bona fide problem in the workplace that he can correct. Demonstrating a cause-and-effect relationship in your report between the sustained injury and workplace conditions can help the safety officer do his job better.

Finally, keep in mind that your workplace is an environment in which you spend a great amount of your time. Your overall health can be adversely affected by workplace conditions, but conversely, if your overall health is good, you may find yourself less vulnerable to injury, especially musculoskeletal injury. Stay fit, stay healthy at home, and you may enjoy a safer, more healthful work experience.

References

1. National Institute for Occupational Safety and Health (NIOSH). 1986. *Proposed National Strategies for the Prevention of Leading Work-Related Diseases and Injuries: Musculoskeletal Injuries*. Cincinnati: NIOSH.
2. American Conference of Governmental Industrial Hygienists. 1997. *ACGIH Today!* 5:5.
3. Ibid.
4. Ozkaya, Nihat, David Goldsheyder and Bernardus Willems. 1996. "Effect of Operator Seat Design on Vibration Exposure." *AIHA Journal* 57:9.
5. Rifkin, Jeremy. 1992. *Beyond Beef: The Rise and Fall of the Cattle Culture*. New York: Dutton.
6. Ibid.
7. Grant, Katharyn A., Daniel J. Habes and Patricia K. Bertsche. 1997. "Lifting Hazards at a Cabinet Manufacturing Company: Evaluation and Recommended Controls." *Applied Occupational and Environmental Hygiene* 12:4.
8. Ibid.
9. Cook, Thomas M., John C. Rosecrance and Chris L. Zimmermann. 1996. "Work-Related Musculoskeletal Disorders in Bricklaying: A Symptom and Job Factors Survey and Guidelines for Improvements." *Applied Occupational and Environmental Hygiene* 11:11.
10. Kelsh, M., H. Morgenstern and D. Ke. 1992. "A Cross-Sectional Study of Carpal Tunnel Syndrome Symptoms Among Trade and Office Workers." *Proceedings of the 9th. International Symposium on Epidemiology in Occupational Health*. Cincinnati: NIOSH.
11. American Industrial Hygiene Association. *The Synergist*. April 15, 1997.
12. Ibid.
13. American Industrial Hygiene Association. *The Synergist*. May/June, 1998.

CHAPTER 11

Do Accidents Happen?

Ellen was not a superstitious person, but every time her husband, Joe, went off to work she said a little prayer for his safety. The construction company that had recently hired him as a crane operator specialized in building highways and Ellen knew the dangers highway workers faced each day, especially in high-traffic areas.

The morning she received a call from the state police she felt her heart jump and something inside told her that Joe was dead. Later, the president of the company called her personally to offer his condolences and to explain to her how rare it was for a crane to topple over. It was a terrible, freak accident that had killed her husband, he said. He told her that she would be receiving a check for $80,000, the payout for accidental death under the state's workers' compensation laws.

It seemed to Ellen a paltry sum to compensate for a man's life, especially when Joe was the sole support of her and her children. He was only 32 when he died. How could anyone compensate her enough for such a grievous loss?

Three days after the accident that changed her life forever, Ellen received a phone call from one of her husband's friends, the man who had gotten Joe his job and who now felt terrible about his death.

"Ellen," the man said, "it was no accident."

"What do you mean? The crane fell over. Everyone saw it happen."

"Yes, but it didn't have to happen. There were no safety supports for the crane. That's why it fell."

Ellen was speechless. Did the company care so little for her husband's safety that they couldn't be bothered adhering to regulations that could have saved his life?

"Ellen, you need to get a lawyer and talk with the Occupational Safety and Health Administration."

What she and her attorney discovered in talking with the local Occupational Safety and Health Administration (OSHA) representative infuriated her. Nine fatalities in the last two years gave the company one of the worst safety records in the state. In the past, the company had been cited by OSHA for several "willful violations" and had been fined over $90,000 by the agency.

Ellen's attorney talked with the survivors of the other company men killed in accidents and organized a class action suit against the company. Together with the state prosecutor's office, her attorney investigated the possibility of bringing criminal manslaughter charges against company executives.

She knew that none of this would bring Joe back to her, but Ellen believed that obtaining justice for him would keep his memory alive, and just possibly save some other family from heartbreak.

Traumatic injuries pose the major threat to the health and well-being of American workers. The National Institute of Occupational Safety and Health (NIOSH) estimates that at least 10 million workers suffer traumatic injuries on the job each year.[1] The Bureau of Labor Statistics' *Census of Occupational Fatalities* survey for 1997 estimated that there were 5,001 workplace fatalities through accidents that year: 14 workers killed each day.[2]

Injuries and deaths due to workplace accidents have devastating effects upon the friends and loved ones of these workers, effects that cannot be measured only in terms of medical costs or workers' compensation. There is no way to measure the effects of the life changes Ellen experienced as a result of the death of her husband, nor is there any way to understand the pain and despair of a young worker who is maimed on the job, with many years of a once productive life snatched away from him.

Yes, tragic, you might say, but accidents happen, right? Despite all the best preventive measures we can employ, workplace accidents will occur and workers will be killed or maimed. The question to ask, though, is how many of these workplace accidents are occurring *needlessly*? How many of them could be avoided by better safety training, safer equipment, and improved workplace conditions and practices?

A more ominous question to ask is how many of these accidents are the result of a company's negligence? How many lives are ruined by a company's willful violation of safety and health regulations, in order to improve its bottom line?

The American workforce's right to a safe and healthful workplace is fully protected by law. Too often, though, the law is violated, someone is killed or seriously injured, and the company goes unpunished, free to do it all over again.

The Problem

Occupational traumatic injuries include amputations, bone breaks and fractures, eye losses, acute poisonings, severe lacerations, and burns. Immediate death is sometimes the result of severe occupational trauma.

In addition to their human toll, occupational traumatic injuries have a devastating effect on the productivity of the U.S. economy and result in astronomical costs. This increased cost of business is always passed on to the consumer.

"Aside from the tragic cost in human suffering to victims and their families, the costs of workplace injuries in dollars are staggering," said Jerry Scannell, president of the National Safety Council. "The total cost is equal to the combined 1996 profits of the twenty largest corporations in America. Companies need to make safety a value in their workplace. Not only do effective safety programs save lives, they're also good business."[3]

In 1997, occupational injuries and deaths cost the U.S. economy $130.7 billion, according to the National Safety Council.[4] This figure included direct costs such as wage losses, insurance costs, and medical costs, and indirect costs such as time lost by other workers and administrative costs connected to investigating and reporting injuries.

There are three variables to consider when investigating the causes of workplace accidents: the workplace, the worker, and the machine.

By the workplace we mean all aspects of the physical environment surrounding a worker on the job that may result in some accidental injury. Wet floors, loose railings and steps, flammable materials, dimly lit areas, vehicular traffic (for roadbuilders, especially), and extreme heat or cold are all workplace sources of potential accidents. The physical environment is the most amenable to corrective action. The hazards are visible and identifiable and are often not difficult to correct.

In addition to the workplace, we must consider the worker himself. The usual factors of age, gender, physical condition, overall health, and incidence of drug or alcohol usage all play a role in how "accident prone" a worker on the job may be. Other factors to be considered are whether or not the worker adheres to all safety policies, uses the recommended safety devices, and has been adequately trained in identifying safety hazards and working in a safe manner. It may not be as easy to discover a worker's personal injury risk as it is to discover workplace hazards. Personal physical conditions that might make the worker more vulnerable to accident may not be easily detected, especially in regard to drug and alcohol use. Also, if an accident occurs and there are no witnesses, it could be difficult to determine whether or not the worker was obeying safety procedures and using safety devices. There is the possibility that the worker will be less than truthful about his own culpability, especially if he was in violation of the company's safety policies.

Finally, we need to consider the machine, the equipment that is being used. Outdated machinery that does not have newer safety devices built in may be a hazard to a worker's safety. The same would apply to machinery that is in poor repair and subject to breakdown. We should consider, too, whether or not the machine is being used properly and for the appropriate task; a welder's torch is not the safest way to warm up coffee during a work break.

Statistics show that the industries with the highest numbers of workplace fatalities include mining, construction, transportation, materials handlers, communications, public utilities, farming, forestry, and fishing. As you would imagine, these industries are also among the highest in the numbers of nonfatal traumatic injuries.

The National Traumatic Occupational Fatalities' surveillance system was developed by OSHA to better understand workplace fatalities by providing a census of occupational injury deaths for all U.S. workers. The surveillance system found that the leading causes of death in the workplace through injury were motor vehicle crashes (23 percent), machine-related incidents (14 percent), homicides (12 percent), falls (10 percent), electrocutions (7 percent), and being struck by falling objects (7 percent).[5]

The construction industry is one of the most dangerous in terms of traumatic injuries and fatalities. In 1995, there were 476,000 nonfatal injuries in the industry, a rate of over 10 per 100 full-time workers. There are many causes of construction site injuries, including vehicular accidents, explosions, trips, lacerations, falls from elevations, and trench cave-ins. The last two are particularly common and deadly.

OSHA's *Excavations* is a 24-page guide to the agency's trenching standard that specifies how trenches for utility and waterlines or foundations must be constructed in order to prevent cave-ins. Cave-ins are a serious problem; former OSHA acting assistant secretary Gregory R. Watchman said, "Though there has been an overall reduction in these types of cases, we continue to be concerned because trenching remains one of the most hazardous operations in the construction industry."[6]

In 1997, OSHA issued citations with proposed penalties totaling $230,400 against Atlantic Contracting, Inc., of Alburtis, Pennsylvania, for subjecting workers to potential life-threatening conditions during installation of a sewer line. The company was charged with 11 alleged violations, 5 of which were alleged to be "willful," after complaints from local residents who had been observing the trenching operation.[7]

Speaking about the citations and the fact that Atlantic Contracting had been cited on three separate occasions, Secretary of Labor Alexis M. Herman said, "Every American has the right to a safe and healthy workplace, and one of my top priorities is to make that right a reality.

We cannot allow employers to continuously place their employees at risk of death or serious injury by ignoring good safety and health practices. By repeatedly endangering its employees' lives, Atlantic brought these penalties on itself."[8]

There are two interesting aspects of the Atlantic Contracting case. The first is that OSHA's inspections resulted from three reports of unsafe work practices received from local citizens. It is encouraging to know that local citizens—who were neither Atlantic workers nor did they have any connection to the workers—were able to take action that may have saved lives and that they were able to take such action without appealing to the courts or their local political representatives. Their action should serve as an example to people who are interested in protecting our workers but who may feel there is no feasible way for them to do so.

The second point worth noting is that OSHA visited the work site on six different occasions in order to acquire proper abatement. Only when all their measures failed did the agency cite Atlantic Contracting.

"The company chose not only to ignore the trenching and excavation standards, but our on-site assistance as well. There simply is no excuse for this blatant disregard for worker safety and flagrant indifference to the law, particularly when assistance is offered," Watchman said.[9]

While OSHA will offer assistance to any industry that is looking for help with occupational safety and health issues, it is unrealistic to think that the agency has the capabilities to monitor all workplaces and make them safe. As long as OSHA remains inadequately funded, it will never have the resources to accomplish this goal. How then can we protect the health and safety of our workers?

One way is to encourage manufacturers of equipment and tools to produce safer products and to mandate those changes if necessary, similar to what was done in the automotive industry to provide seat belts and air bags. Farm tractors are an example of how this might work to protect workers.

Farmer Jones, working in the American hinterlands, will probably never see an OSHA inspector in his lifetime. Jones has been farming his land for 30 years, his farming skills taught to him by his father, who learned them from his father, and so on. There isn't anything Jones doesn't know about farming, including the safety risks of using a variety of equipment, and he doesn't need any Washington bureaucrat telling him how to do his job. He knows that accidents happen on a farm—it's part of the job—and there isn't much anyone can do about that. He knows there wasn't anything he could have done when his father's old tractor rolled over on the bank of a drainage ditch, crushing him to death; Jones still uses that same tractor.

Tractor rollovers account for about half of all fatalities involving farm tractors; an Iowa study over the five-year period from 1988 to 1992 indicated that 15 overturn fatalities occurred each year.[10] It is estimated that the yearly costs from deaths from tractor overturns in Iowa are a minimum of $3.78 million. This is based on lost income potential only and does not include hidden costs nor the costs of disabling injuries.

In 1965, some tractor manufacturers began building tractors with rollover protective structures, a cab or frame that protects the operator—along with seat belts—from being crushed by the tractor if the machine should roll over. In 1985, tractor manufacturers adopted a voluntary standard to sell *all* tractors with rollover protective structures in place. As a result of the manufacturers' actions, any farmer buying a tractor built in 1985 or after is automatically protected by rollover protective structures (as long as he keeps the structure in place). There is no doubt that these tractors are more expensive than older models without rollover protective structures and that the extra cost is passed on to the farmer buying the machine, but the extra cost up front could save the farmer money in the form of lost productivity as a result of a tractor injury and could even save his life.

Still, many tractors made more than 40 years ago, like Farmer Jones's, are still operational today; it is estimated that fewer than one-third of the 4.4 million tractors used for agricultural purposes have rollover protective structures in place.[11] Since it is these older tractors that are most involved in accidents, tractor rollovers will continue to be a source of accidents for farmers until the machines are finally phased out of service and replaced by newer models.

Building safer equipment will help save workers' lives and prevent accidents, but there also needs to be an increased awareness of safety issues among workers. They need to develop a greater perception of their risks in their workplaces and learn how to minimize those risks. It is interesting to note that in an Iowa Farm and Rural Life poll of 2,016 Iowa farm families, farmers indicated that they perceived insecticides as the most hazardous item they worked with and tractors as the least hazardous. Yet, for those farmers who reported having had an accident, farm machinery was the number one item involved—with tractors being fourth—while no acute accidents involving insecticides were reported.[12] Better safety and health education is an important step in helping workers to develop an accurate perception of the dangers inherent in their workplaces.

What Can Be Done?

The U.S. Public Health Service in its lengthy report *Healthy People 2000: National Health Promotion and Disease*

Prevention Objectives has established the following goals to improve occupational safety and health by the year 2000: to reduce work-related fatalities through injuries to no more than 4 per 100,000 workers (a 33 percent decrease); to reduce work-related injuries to no more than 6 per 100 workers (a 22 percent decrease).[13]

What can be done to reduce traumatic injuries and fatalities in the workplace and to help achieve these goals? A 1996 report developed by NIOSH's National Occupational Research Agenda Traumatic Injury Team outlines a model for researching and reducing traumatic injuries in the workplace. The elements of this model include:

- **Injury surveillance**—This refers to the collection, analysis, and interpretation of data on injuries, hazards, and exposures, with the goal of identifying potential risk factors for further research, and for prevention planning and intervention evaluation.
- **Analytic injury research**—This research attempts to quantify and prioritize risk factors. In addition to statistical data other, nontraditional research methods are used, including the analysis of social, cultural, and economic characteristics of industries and work sites.
- **Prevention and control**—Occupational injury control requires a multidimensional approach, including education, engineering, and enforcement efforts; any single strategy may not be sufficiently effective, but when combined can result in substantial reductions in occupational injuries.
- **Communication/dissemination/technology transfer**—One of the principal factors affecting the reduction of occupational injuries is the effective organization and communication of knowledge and technology related to occupational risks and prevention. Knowledge and technology developed through research must be communicated or transferred to employers, workers, and

others who can apply this information to prevent injuries.

- **Evaluation**—Monitoring and evaluating the results of intervention efforts is essential in determining the effectiveness of those interventions. Although many intervention programs have been established in the workplace, few of them have undergone rigorous evaluation to determine their effectiveness.

What can you do specifically to protect yourself from workplace injuries? First, as always, know everything you can about your workplace and the materials and equipment you use. Consider the adage that knowledge is power and remember that the knowledge you possess about your job may empower you to be accident-free.

Next, try to maintain a realistic perception of the risks in your workplace and assess how you structure your job tasks relative to that perception. As an example, common sense may warn you not to walk under a scaffold without a hard hat, but you've been on the job for five months and you've not seen so much as a single nail fall from one. What are the odds that a hammer would fall just as you walked by? An accurate perception of the risks in your workplace would tell you that there is *always* the chance, no matter how remote, of a falling hammer.

Third, always follow safety procedures to the last detail and always use whatever safety equipment is recommended for your job. Maybe the task takes a little longer if you're using safety equipment that may encumber you slightly, but the extra time could possibly save your life.

Finally, it is important that you fill out an incident report as accurately as possible should you be injured on the job (if your employer does not use incident reports, you might consider asking him to start). It is important that your supervisor accurately record what happened and not simply write up the accident as "employee error."

Only by understanding the causes of accidents can future ones be prevented. Careful study of such reports can help occupational safety and health officers better identify and understand occupational risks and will help them formulate corrective actions and intervention programs that will protect you.

References

1. National Institute for Occupational Safety and Health (NIOSH). 1986. *Proposed National Strategies for the Prevention of Leading Work-Related Diseases and Injuries: Severe Occupational Traumatic Injuries.* Cincinnati: NIOSH.
2. National Safety Council. 1998. *Safety + Health* May.
3. American Conference of Governmental Industrial Hygienists. 1997. *ACGIH Today!* 5:6.
4. National Safety Council. 1998. *Safety + Health* May.
5. National Institute for Occupational Safety and Health (NIOSH). 1993. *Fatal Injuries to Workers in the United States, 1980–1989: A Decade of Surveillance.* Cincinnati: NIOSH.
6. Occupational Safety and Health Administration (OSHA). 1997. Internet *OSHA News Release* August 27.
7. Ibid.
8. Ibid.
9. Ibid.
10. National Institute for Occupational Safety and Health (NIOSH). 1996. *Trac-Safe: A Community-Based Program for Reducing Injuries and Deaths from Tractor Overturns.* Cincinnati: NIOSH.
11. Ibid.
12. Ibid.
13. Department of Health and Human Services. 1990. *Healthy People 2000: National Health Promotion and Disease Prevention Objectives.* Washington: U.S. Government Printing Office.

CHAPTER 12

In Pursuit of Justice

There are very few of us who are not aware of the destruction that technology and progress has wreaked upon our natural environment. Whether we are talking about damaging the ozone layer, poisoning the rivers and oceans, or cutting down the rain forests, the debate over environmental damage has been widespread and grows ever more vocal. While much remains to be done to protect the fragile natural environment, progress is being made. The world's public consciousness has been touched, and, if knowledgeable and well-meaning folks prevail, we will find a way to protect what is left of our natural world and, perhaps, recover what has seemingly been lost.

Millions of us, however, will continue to spend most of our waking lives in a workplace environment that can adversely affect our health and well-being. We must give serious thought to the unsafe and unhealthful conditions that characterize the workplace and strive to change them; future generations may thank us for cleaner water, but they will chide us for failing to reduce the prevalence of occupational disease.

It is entirely within our capabilities to create a safe and healthful workplace. This may not happen overnight, but it *can* happen. We have only to resolve to use the legal, economic, and technological means at our disposal to create such a working environment.

Beyond Self-Protection

We have already shown that many workers lose their lives on the job, either immediately as in workplace accidents, or, much later in life, as a result of a workplace-induced disease. It could be argued that these workers knew the dangers their jobs entailed and that they had the freedom to leave them at any time and find work elsewhere. Many workers do just that, but for some, that is simply not an option. Not every worker has the luxury of throwing off one job for another, especially if that worker is largely unskilled, undereducated, past his working prime, or a minority (either gender or race). For these workers, adverse health effects in the workplace simply become part of their lives.

But is it right that workers should be forced to give up their jobs, their careers, because of unhealthful workplace conditions? Shouldn't the emphasis be on creating healthful workplaces rather than insisting that workers, if they want to continue working, meekly accept dangerous conditions as "part of the job"?

We have already shown various ways through which workers can educate themselves about the safety and health of their workplaces and we have provided practical information that will help many workers better protect themselves from unhealthful and unsafe conditions at work. Still, there is only so much any worker can do to protect himself; much of the burden for creating a safe and healthful workplace lies with the corporation.

Most American corporations understand the value of a contented workforce and do what they can to keep their employees happy. A safe and healthful workplace is usually thought of as one way to maintain a satisfied workforce. Most companies understand the value and intent of safety and health regulations and try to comply with the Occupational Safety and Health Administration's (OSHA) standards.

There are, of course, exceptions to this way of thinking. There are some corporations who try to skimp on safety and health practices, sometimes in order to save money, sometimes as a reaction to what is seen as governmental bureaucracy interfering in business. The degree to which these companies flout safety and health regulations will vary and the violations may not be all that serious. In such corporations, labor unions or concerned employees may be able to ensure the corporation's compliance to safety and health regulations without too much effort; a single letter from OSHA, based on an employee complaint, may do the trick.

Then there are the truly dangerous corporations, those few that will not allow safety and health regulations to stand in the way of their profits. These corporations believe occupational illness, accidents, or fatalities to be merely part of the cost of doing business. A review of OSHA files would show that many of these companies are repeat offenders; they frequently refuse to comply with OSHA regulations and are fined repeatedly as they ignore orders for corrective action. Thankfully, there are not many such corporations in the United States.

There needs to be a change in the way we think about work and how we see ourselves fitting into the workplace. Workers must recognize not only the economic value they represent to their employers, but their own personal value as well, their dignity and integrity, their health and well-being. There should not have to be a choice between a worker's well-being and corporate success, but if that choice is demanded, the well-being of the worker must take precedence.

Making that choice is not always easy, however. It is

OSHA's policy that a certain number of workplace deaths are "acceptable"; that is, any given safety standard that the agency has established is based upon striking a balance between worker safety and health and the demands of the corporate world for profits. The corporations cite the expenses incurred in setting up safety procedures and may even threaten to relocate overseas or go out of business entirely because they cannot afford the price of making their workplaces safer. So, OSHA works out a compromise with business and enacts a standard based on cost-benefit analysis, a standard that the agency knows will result in a certain number of deaths, an "acceptable" number.

To be fair to OSHA, none of the agency's standards can become law without the approval of Congress. As you would expect, this brings into play political favors, paybacks, payoffs, and corporate lobbying. In other words, the merits of the proposed standard may take a backseat to political expediency and patronage. In most cases, OSHA is lucky to get any standards enacted at all. Can anyone wonder why the agency might settle for acceptable deaths and the less-than-perfect standard in lieu of no standard at all?

Even when rigid OSHA regulations are in effect, some companies ignore them. This book has shown numerous cases of workplace-induced disease, injury, and death, some of which occur with the full knowledge and the tacit acceptance of the corporations. How can this happen?

According to our legal system, a criminal act is criminal only if it is intended to be so and the accused possesses the mental state to understand his intentions. The legal term that refers to the mental state of the accused is *mens rea*. This rules out harmful acts that are accidents, since the intent to do harm is absent. The *mens rea* argument has been the linchpin of many a corporation's defense against criminal charges, no matter what those charges were. The corporation does not have a mind, corporate lawyers would argue, it is not a thinking, rational being. Therefore, how can it ever have the intention to do harm?

This argument has not been easy for prosecutors to overcome. In cases where they have been successful in prosecuting a case, lawyers have been able to prove *mens rea* among the corporation's policymakers, the collective knowledge of all its employees, or the corporation's own expressed or implied policies. While these arguments have allowed some cases to proceed against corporations, it is an extremely rare case that results in little more than fines for the offending corporation. The fines are usually so paltry compared to the corporation's financial assets that the company considers them simply the cost of doing business, equivalent to some licensing fee necessary to carry out its business. Note well that it is the corporation that is sentenced, and not an *individual* within the corporation.

Criminal prosecutions under the Occupational Safety and Health Act of 1970, the congressional act that created OSHA, are rare since they are reserved for egregious situations in which a worker is killed on the job as a result of a company's "willful violation" of a safety and health standard. The act relies on civil actions for violations rather than on criminal prosecution. It is up to state and federal prosecutors to implement criminal prosecution for charges such as assault and battery, manslaughter, and homicide.

Even when a corporation is found guilty of criminal activity relative to workplace diseases or fatalities, it is not found guilty of assault, manslaughter, or homicide, as one would expect, but is found guilty of other acts that revolve around the actual crimes against its workers. For instance, it may be found guilty of perjury, jury tampering, destroying evidence, perhaps fraud or conspiracy, as the company tries to cover up the true crime or somehow minimize its import, but never anything as serious as murder. Once again, it is usually the difficulty in establishing *mens rea* that works in favor of the defendant.

An example of this is the case of Manville, formerly the nation's largest asbestos manufacturer, and the incidence of asbestosis among workers who handle asbestos products (and even their families who inhale asbestos fibers from the clothing of the worker when he returns home).[1] For decades, Manville had been shipping its asbestos products to shipyards, factories, construction sites, and other industries without labels warning of the dangers of inhaling the substance. There were no warning labels on their products, nor were their workers informed of the dangers of asbestos despite the fact that asbestos disease was reported as early as 1908.

As more workers became aware of the health danger posed by asbestos, they began to speak out, with many of them bringing forth workers' compensation claims. In a 1978 congressional hearing on asbestos, internal documents from the asbestos industry became public. It was clear from these documents that the industry had engaged in cover-ups and denials in an attempt to downplay the dangers of asbestos. The documents were reviewed by James Price, a judge from South Carolina, who said that they demonstrated "a pattern of denial and disease and attempts at suppression of information."[2] Particularly damning to Manville's claim of ignorance was the fact that the company had settled eleven compensation cases out of court in 1933 despite the fact that Manville said it first recognized the dangers of asbestos in 1964.

The documents also revealed that asbestos company executives had strong-armed industry publications into refraining from publishing damaging health studies and that the asbestos companies themselves had banded together to fund their own studies, which, not surprisingly, showed asbestos to be less of a health problem than industry detractors said it was.

In the wake of the congressional hearings, personal injury lawsuits against the asbestos industry escalated; by 1984 there were more than 25,000 pending suits with 500 new cases being filed every month. The claimed damages totaled hundreds of millions of dollars.

In 1982 Manville filed for bankruptcy in order to protect itself from the personal injury suits lodged against it. After three years of legal maneuvering, Manville agreed to pay $2.5 billion to thousands of claimants. The company set up a fund to which shareholders gave up half their stock. In addition, much of Manville's projected earnings over the next 25 years would go to the fund. No one individual, from Manville or any other asbestos company, was ever held criminally liable for his actions.

But there have been some successful criminal prosecutions for safety and health violations. In 1992 Emmet J. Roe, owner of Imperial Foods in Hamlet, North Carolina, was sentenced to nearly twenty years in prison after pleading guilty to involuntary manslaughter for a fire at his chicken-processing plant the year before in which twenty-five workers died. As part of his plea bargain, all charges were dropped against his son (the company's operations manager) and the plant manager.[3]

The January 28, 1998, edition of the *San Francisco Chronicle* reported that the owner of an Oakland, California, electroplating plant in which a worker died in a toxic vat and a neighborhood was threatened by a potentially catastrophic leak had agreed to serve up to one year in jail and pay as much as $200,000 in fines.[4]

While we can do everything in our power to protect our health and safety on the job, there are some measures that should be taken to ensure that corporations are held liable for any willful actions that endanger their workers' health.

First, it is important that corporations should not enjoy the same legal rights as individuals, such as the right to a jury trial, and the rights of privacy and freedom from self-incrimination. These individual rights were established in order to protect a person from the strength of legal authorities in a court of law and to allow him a better chance of defending himself. When a rich and powerful corporation is on trial, it can marshal more legal firepower than the authorities prosecuting it and is in little danger of being overwhelmed by them. If anything, exactly the opposite takes place and the local prosecutor finds himself facing a battery of high-powered corporate lawyers in the courtroom and might also find himself being maneuvered outside the courtroom by politicians, businessmen, and lobbyists, all of whom may have a personal stake in the company. Even a skilled and competent prosecutor can be bowled over by such unrelenting pressure.

Second, corporate executives must be forced to take responsibility for their actions. Legislation needs to be enacted at the federal level that would make executives liable for corporate actions that injure or kill workers. Passing a law of executive responsibility, though, is not necessarily the same thing as finding an executive guilty of criminal acts such as assault or homicide. Since a company's activities often cut across state and international boundaries, a federal law needs to be enacted in which corporations and their executives may be tried for homicide. Some state prosecutors have brought forth these charges with little consequence, but a federal law allows other agencies, with more muscle than a state prosecutor, to enter the fray and make the charges stick.

Third, we must lobby to make sure that the safety and

health policing agencies such as OSHA, the Environmental Protection Agency (EPA), and the Food and Drug Administration (FDA) have the manpower and the budgets necessary to do their jobs correctly. That has not been the case recently and some presidents, notably Ronald Reagan, have cut allocations to these agencies way back in a none too subtle effort to prevent their "interfering" with business.

OSHA has only 924 inspectors, responsible for 90 million workers at 7 million worksites. This means the agency can inspect workplaces on average every 109 years. Obviously, with so few inspectors in the workplace, serious safety and health violations often go undetected. An adequate budget would allow OSHA to do its job much more efficiently.

Fourth, workers must be able to notify the proper authorities of safety and health violations in the workplace without fear of reprisal from their employers. Workers can bring complaints to OSHA or the National Institute for Occupational Safety and Health (NIOSH) anonymously except that their complaint must be specific and that specificity means that the company can often deduce who actually lodged the complaint. As an example, if you file a complaint with OSHA about a paint-spraying booth in your workplace, and you are one of the two workers in that area, there is a pretty good chance your supervisor will find out that you filed the complaint. Also, you probably went to OSHA or NIOSH as a last resort, and only after you had already complained to your supervisor through the proper corporate channels without the problem being corrected; now you are on record as being a complainer and any activity from OSHA or NIOSH could be easily traced back to you.

While the federal government has laws to protect whistle-blowers who work for the government (some states have similar laws) there needs to be much greater protection for whistle-blowers nationwide, in both the public and private sectors. Workers must be able to report criminal violations in the workplace without fear of being sued or losing their jobs.

Finally, sentences for convicted corporate executives must have some teeth to them. A convicted executive should be required to serve appropriate time in prison for his crimes, should be fined an amount that is actually punitive, and should be made to pay restitution to his victims. None of these actions are being taken with any great deal of success currently. For instance, a violation of the Occupational Safety and Health Act that results in a fatality carries a maximum penalty of a $10,000 fine and six months in prison. You could spend more time in jail for stealing a Mars bar from your local 7-Eleven.

The Chink in the Armor

We said earlier that corporations, or their executives, are rarely convicted of assault, manslaughter, or homicide relative to workplace diseases, injuries, and deaths. It is more likely that they would be convicted of other, less serious charges related to the crime, such as perjury, destroying evidence, or conspiracy. Still, there is some hope that some of these more serious charges may stick in future cases. Some attempts have already been made.

In the summer of 1998, a grand jury charged LeMaster Steel Erectors Inc. of Indiana with one count of willfully violating federal safety regulations and three counts of obstructing justice in a case involving the death of one of its workers who died from a fall two years prior.[5]

"This is the first time in the history of OSHA that we have obtained an indictment against a company for obstruction of justice," said Cincinnati-area OSHA director William Murphy.[6]

It may have been the first time an obstruction of justice charge was ever filed, but it was not the first time LeMaster had been in trouble with OSHA. The company had been cited several times for failing to provide adequate safety precautions for its employees who were exposed to dangers of falling from steel structures. As part of resolving their problems with OSHA, the company agreed to develop a fall-protection system that should have been in place when the worker was killed.

The obstruction of justice charges revolved around a LeMaster foreman who allegedly lied to OSHA officials and told them that safety cables were in place when the worker fell and who then had them installed immediately after the accident. A company supervisor was also charged with obstruction of justice by allegedly telling witnesses to the accident not to reveal the lack of fall protection. In October 1998, additional charges of conspiracy to obstruct justice, commit perjury, and defraud the United States in order to conceal the true condition of safety equipment at the accident site were brought against the company. The company safety officer was also indicted for conspiracy and lying to a grand jury.

LeMaster pleaded innocent and the case is still pending as this book is written, but the company could be fined $500,000 on each of the four counts of obstructing justice, if convicted. The foreman, supervisor, and safety officer could possibly receive jail time if they are convicted.

Speaking about the LeMaster case, the assistant secretary of labor for occupational safety and health and the head of OSHA, Charles N. Jeffress, said: "The indictments returned today in Ohio emphasize the importance of worker safety in our country. We want to assist employers in providing that safety for their employees. However, during the course of our investigations, we will not hesitate to refer a case to the Department of Justice for possible criminal prosecution, if we believe it's warranted. That is precisely what happened with LeMaster."[7]

In light of how few corporate executives have ever faced criminal charges for workplace diseases, accidents, and fatalities, it's encouraging to hear such tough talk from the OSHA administrator. Sometimes, that tough talk has been backed up by significant fines levied against corporations by OSHA, but some cases make you wonder whether they are enough.

As an example, in 1998 OSHA proposed fines totaling $463,024 against the Claremont Steel Corporation of Claremont, New Hampshire.[8] Two workers had been using a hydraulic jack, positioned between two, 62-foot-long steel beams, to try to bend and shape them. The jack slipped out and the two workers were killed instantly when the beams slammed together.

An OSHA investigation revealed that the jack had been damaged earlier and so did not properly hold the load. It was discovered that another employee had been injured earlier due to a slipping jack. OSHA ordered that any damaged jacks still in service be removed immediately. Almost two weeks after the fatal accident, an OSHA inspector found another damaged jack in use.

Most of the huge fine OSHA levied against Claremont was for ten "willful violations," violations in which a corporation says, in effect, "we know that what we are doing is against the law but, frankly, we just don't give a damn." (Claremont was also charged with seventy other violations of a less serious nature; as this book is being written, the Occupational Safety and Health Review Commission is reviewing litigation between Claremont and OSHA.)

In 1996, a ten-foot-deep trench collapsed, killing one worker and seriously injuring two others in Margate, Florida.[9] The men, employees of Richard E. Fowler, Inc., had been laying water and sewer lines in the trench when it caved in, burying them beneath a heavy chunk of compacted soil and gravel. The OSHA investigation showed that there had been minor cave-ins earlier in the day and that several people at the job site had notified the employer of the dangerous trench condition. Still, nothing was done to protect the men in the trench.

OSHA initially proposed fines for ten violations against Fowler in the amount of $448,000.

"Because of Fowler's blatant disregard for his employees' safety, we are proposing the maximum possible penalty in this case," said then acting assistant secretary for occupational safety and health Gregory R. Watchman. "Let there be no doubt: when workers' lives are at stake, their safety must come first—not profits or deadlines or convenience."[10] Fowler contested the OSHA citations but they were upheld, although reduced to $350,000.

Throughout this book we have shown how workers can protect themselves in the workplace. We have also demonstrated the many things corporations can do to protect the safety and health of their workers. A truly safe workplace can come about only through the cooperation of the corporation with its workers. Most companies play by the rules and comply as best they can with existing safety and health regulations, but some do not. For workers in those companies, there must be legal recourse that allows them to protect themselves. The legal consequences for the corporation must be severe and punitive. The law must treat corporations and corporate executives as criminals when the offenses warrant such a label and the prosecution must be swift, decisive, and equitable to the crime.

References

1. Mokhiber, Russell. 1989. *Corporate Crime and Violence: Big Business Power and the Abuse of the Public Trust.* San Francisco: Sierra Club Books.
2. Ibid.
3. *Sojourners.* December, 1992.
4. Sarvadi J.D., CIH, David G. May. 1998. "Criminal Prosecution Under the OSHA Act." *Compliance Magazine.*
5. *The Cincinnati Enquirer,* July 16, 1998.
6. Ibid.
7. Occupational Safety and Health Administration. July 15, 1998. Internet OSHA *News Release.*
8. Occupational Safety and Health Administration. May 28, 1998. Internet OSHA *News Release.* May 28.
9. Occupational Safety and Health Administration. April 30, 1997. Internet OSHA *News Release.*
10. Ibid.

CHAPTER 13

Getting Help

Thus far, this book has attempted to demonstrate the extent and severity of safety and health risks prevalent in the American workplace. Although we have tried to use a wide variety of examples to illustrate our point, it is impossible to speak of the dangers of every occupation or every work site in a single book. It is our hope, however, that even if a reader did not read about his particular occupation, he at least would come away with an awareness of the magnitude of workplace safety and health issues and that he would become more observant of possible risks in his own workplace. This final chapter will help readers who are concerned about workplace safety and health and are looking for a way to improve their workplaces.

Where Do I Go?

Let's assume that you have discovered some type of safety and health risk in your workplace—perhaps you've linked that persistent neck pain to the position of your computer monitor, or you've noticed that your skin itches and blisters as you launder patients' sheets in the hospital laundry, or you've observed how oily the floor is in the brake repair shop and you worry about slipping on it. In any case, you've discovered a health risk and you would like it corrected. What do you do?

We do not recommend that you complain to a state or federal agency as your first course of action. It is very possible that the workplace risk you have discovered may be easily corrected and that your employer would be amenable to doing so. Use the proper channels within your company to make your concerns known. These may include a supervisor, a union steward, a safety officer or committee, the human resources director, the suggestion box, etc. Let your employer know about the problem and ask what can be done to correct it. Proposing a possible solution yourself may help in getting the problem corrected.

Suppose you take your concerns to the proper authorities in your company and they fail to do anything about them. What then?

At this point, you have the right to contact either the Occupational Safety and Health Administration (OSHA) or the National Institute for Occupational Safety and Health (NIOSH) and ask them to look into the matter. It is important to remember that both agencies will respond to anonymous complaints but that there is always the possibility of your employer discovering the source of the complaint. You must determine for yourself whether or not you are willing to take that risk.

OSHA and NIOSH have very different responsibilities and their responses to complaints will be different, so it is important to understand how each agency works and where their focus lies.

OSHA—As we have stated before, OSHA is the occupational safety and health "policeman." It is the agency's job to investigate suspected violations of occupational safety and health laws and to take the appropriate legal action to correct violations of those laws.

You may contact OSHA anonymously and ask the

agency to investigate your concern. The agency is not required to visit your workplace and investigate it, however, limited as the agency is by inadequate staffing and funding. It is more likely that an OSHA officer will send a letter (the letter will not reveal your name if you requested anonymity) to your employer telling him that the agency has received a complaint and asking your employer for a response. Depending upon the response OSHA receives from your employer, they may pursue the case or not.

If your complaint is serious, and OSHA perceives it as a problem in which they have a particular interest, or your employer's response letter is unsatisfactory, they may visit your work site. OSHA inspectors do not have to announce their arrival beforehand and by law have the right to enter the work site, even if it takes a warrant to do so. While on-site, the inspectors will investigate your specific complaint but are also free to check any other suspected safety and health violations that may exist. For these reasons, companies do not generally welcome visits from OSHA and will try to ward off such visits by a well-crafted reply to the original OSHA letter, sometimes using inaccurate or dishonest responses, such as stating that they have already corrected the problem when in fact they have just started work on it.

OSHA may issue citations and levy fines against your employer for any safety and health violations the investigators discover. The company may appeal these fines and get them dismissed or reduced. However, depending upon when OSHA starts its clock, fines can be levied on a daily basis, so they will increase as time goes by without corrective actions.

In the last several years, OSHA has been designing programs to encourage industry's voluntary compliance with safety and health regulations. The agency has agreed to suspend routine inspections to some businesses that are voluntarily working to correct safety and health problems and are keeping OSHA informed of their progress. OSHA has also targeted some industries with poor safety and health records for regular inspections, in the hopes of encouraging these industries to participate more actively in correcting them.

OSHA is also working with the Small Business Administration to provide safety and health consultants to small businesses who are trying to create safe workplaces. These consultants are not OSHA compliance officers and do not have the authority to issue citations.

NIOSH—Unlike OSHA, NIOSH will not act on a complaint unless three employees, the employer, or a labor union file it (it may be filed anonymously). The primary difference between NIOSH and OSHA is that any action taken by NIOSH on your behalf will not result in citations or fines and your employer will not be required to correct the problem, although NIOSH will send a copy of its report to the local OSHA office. This is because NIOSH is a research organization only and has no law enforcement abilities.

When NIOSH receives a complaint, agency officers review it and decide if it is appropriate for the agency to investigate. Generally, NIOSH is interested in researching new or poorly understood safety and health issues and will not involve itself with problems that can be easily corrected by an industrial hygienist.

If NIOSH decides to investigate your complaint, a team of researchers will come out and conduct scientific monitoring and evaluations of your workplace. They will then write a report that may take months or even years to complete, in which they publish the research team's findings. This report would be available from NIOSH's publications department to anyone who wanted one.

While NIOSH may make recommendations for corrective actions in the report, you must remember that the agency's findings are not binding and are not law. However, when OSHA considers a new safety and health standard, the agency will frequently rely on information obtained by NIOSH as a guide to setting the standard.

A NIOSH report also has the effect of informing the public about a particular safety and health issue, which may result in more complaints, which may then result in OSHA developing a standard (if one is not already in place) and enforcing it.

To help you in finding your way toward creating a safe and healthful workplace, the names, addresses, and contact information for OSHA, NIOSH, and other agencies are listed below. Associations that can provide information on general safety and health issues, as well as the science of industrial hygiene, are also listed.

Resources

American Association of Occupational Health Nurses, Inc.
2920 Brandywine Road, Suite 100
Atlanta, GA 30341
Phone: 770-455-7757
Internet: www.aaohn.org

American Board of Industrial Hygiene
6015 W. St. Joseph, Suite 102
Lansing, MI 48917-3980
Phone: 517-321-2638
Internet: www.abih.org

American Conference of Governmental Industrial Hygienists (ACGIH)
Kemper Woods Center
1330 Kemper Meadow Dr., Suite 600
Cincinnati, OH 45240-1634
Phone: 513-742-2020
Internet: www.acgih.org

American Industrial Hygiene Association (AIHA)
2700 Prosperity Avenue, Suite 250
Fairfax, VA 22031
Phone: 703-849-8888
Internet: www.aiha.org

American Public Health Association
1015 15th. St. NW, Suite 300
Washington, DC 20005
Phone: 202-789-5600
Internet: www.apha.org/

Department of Health and Human Services
Health Resources and Services Administration
5600 Fishers Lane
Rockville, MD 20857
Phone: 301-443-2865
Internet: www.dhhs.gov/progorg/oig/

Environmental Protection Agency (EPA)
EPA Publications and Information Center
P.O. Box 42419
Cincinnati, OH 45242-0419
Phone: 800-535-0202
Internet: www.epa.gov

International Occupational Hygiene Association
Suite 2, Georgian House
Great Northern Rd.
Derby
DE1 1LT

United Kingdom
Phone: 011-44-1332-298101
Internet: www.bohs.org/ioha/

Mine Safety and Health Administration
Department of Labor
4015 Wilson Blvd.
Arlington, VA 22203
Phone: 703-235-1452
Internet: www.msha.gov/

National Institute for Occupational Safety and Health (NIOSH)
200 Independence Ave., SW
Washington, DC 20201
Phone: 202-401-0721
Internet: www.cdc.gov/niosh/homepage.html

National Safety Council
1121 Spring Lake Dr.
Itasca, IL 60143-3201
Phone: 630-285-1121
Internet: www.nsc.org/

Occupational Safety and Health Administration (OSHA)
U.S. Department of Labor
200 Constitution Ave., NW
Washington, DC 20210
Phone: 202-219-8151
Emergency: 800-321-OSHA
Internet: www.osha.gov/

World Health Organization
Avenue Appia 20
1211 Geneva 27
Switzerland
Phone: (41-22) 791-21-11
Internet: www.who.int

World Safety Organization
World Management Center
P.O. Box 518, 305 Market St.
Warrensburg, MO 64093
Phone: 660-747-3132
Internet: www. worldsafety.org/

Other Internet Sites of Interest

Bureau of Labor Statistics, Safety and Health Statistics
http://stats.bls.gov/oshhome.htm

Office of Women's Health
www.cdc.gov/od/owh

Indoor Environment Review
www.iaqpubs.com/ier.html

Institute of Occupational Safety Engineering
http: turva24.me.tut.fi/

Women: Work and Health
www.cdc.gov/nchswww

Index